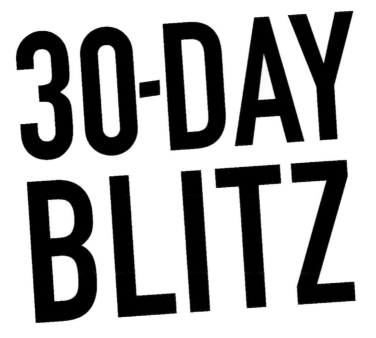

30-DAY BLITZ

CHARLOTTE CROSBY'S

30-DAY BLITZ

WORKOUTS, MEAL PLANS AND OVER 60 RECIPES FOR A BODY YOU'LL LOVE IN LESS THAN A MONTH

HEADLINE

First published in 2017 by HEADLINE PUBLISHING GROUP

1

Cataloguing in Publication Data is available from the British Library

Trade Paperback ISBN 978 1 4722 4331 7

Recipes created by Kat Mead
Exercise programme created by David Souter
Diet plan created by Kerry Torrens
Management by Bold Management
Food photography by Haarala Hamilton
Food styling by Kat Mead
Props styling by Jemima Hetherington

All photographs of Charlotte by Alex James except pages 82 and 189 by Ewelina Stechnij
Hair and make-up by Michael Phillips

Design and art direction by Lynne Eve, Design Jam
Colour reproduction by Born London

Printed and bound in Germany by Firmengruppe APPL

CONTENTS

INTRODUCTION

People always ask me, 'Charlotte what do you eat?' I'm not talking about the sort of question you get when you're invited to dinner at someone's house; I mean people come up to me in the street or tweet me and they want a literal breakdown of what goes into my stomach on a daily basis.

'Give me your diet plan!' they always say, 'I need to follow it step by step!'

Because the truth is, sometimes you don't just want to hear what's healthy for you – you want to know exactly what to eat and exactly when to eat it. And I'm the same – whether it's hair, clothes or make-up – it's so much easier to copy something someone else has already done!

So, in July 2017, I decided to go on social media and tell people what I do. I told them every last detail about what I was eating each day for a week. I told them what exercises I was doing and when I was doing them. The only thing I left out was how often I went to the loo (and most of the time I described that too). I turned it into a challenge and my hashtag was #FOF which stood for 'Fuck Off Fat'. Not really the sort of title that's going to get TV commissioners excited, thinking that this is going to be the next *Great British Bake Off*, but it worked for me!

I was overwhelmed by how many people responded! Hundreds of you joined in and started following the same plan and routine as me. I told everyone to take photos of themselves doing the exercises and send them to me and, all of a sudden, I was being tagged in loads of pictures. I must have been tagged about 18,000 times! I thought, 'Oh my God! What have I started?!' because I was worried I might not be able to keep it up. But I realised it was just me doing the same things I do every day, only this time I was documenting it.

Obviously, there was a bit too much oversharing a couple of times; like when I weighed myself (something I don't think you should do very often because it makes you focus on the wrong goals) and had a moan because I'd put on weight. I was 10 stone 8 and the last time I'd weighed myself I was 9 stone 5, which when you're 5 foot 6 is really slim. It was a stupid thing to moan about as I wasn't overweight for my height – I was well within what's considered 'normal' so it was really irresponsible of me to talk about it in public in that way, and more importantly I looked perfectly good and felt happy with myself. I've always said don't become obsessed with how much you weigh – scales can be so depressing and make you feel like shit. Instead it should be about how you look to yourself and how you feel inside. I really should have followed my own advice.

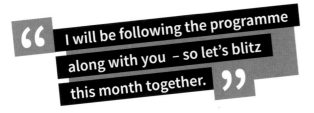

"I will be following the programme along with you – so let's blitz this month together."

So that's how the idea for this book was born! It's a way of sharing all of the stuff I do and eat to get me towards the fittest version of myself. And it's not just about getting fit. This book is as much about making you happy on the inside as the outside. I know it sounds silly but I honestly think that since losing weight (I have managed to keep off three stone since being at my biggest in *Geordie Shore* four years ago) I am a brighter, happier and more positive (well, most of the time) person. Before I learnt what my body needs in terms of food and exercise to look good, I was actually pretty depressed; I just didn't fully realise it. It was only once I shifted the flab that I felt like a new person – I wanted to jump out of bed in the morning and I felt like I could take over the world (so watch out Trump – I'm after your job!).

I read on the Internet that breaking a habit takes 21 days so that's why I've made this book 30 days – because it will make sure you definitely change things and break all your bad habits. Throughout the plan I've given you other challenges to do on the journey to getting yourself fitter and feeling better. And I will be following the programme along with you – so let's blitz this month together. At the end of the 30 days we will both be feeling so much more energetic, healthier, shinier and more positive!

MAKE FRIENDS WITH EXERCISE

Me and Exercise have only really become mates over the last four years. I never liked Exercise. I hated her in fact. I never wanted to hang out with her – she was like the really annoying girl who always asked too many questions. But then I realised there are negative points about every friend and you've just got to accept them for who they are and not neglect them. So, this book is about not neglecting your mate Exercise. It's about a big commitment to the friendship!

Exercise makes you feel so much better about everything else in your life. Think about getting up on a Monday morning feeling sluggish and hating the fact you have to go to work. When you are in your fitness zone and on a mission, if you get up early to do a bit of a workout you will start your week feeling happy and alive and raring to go. You will have energy and happy endorphins will come out of you from every orifice. You will feel so great. It won't feel like a Monday – it will feel like a Saturday! In fact, every day on my 30-Day Blitz will be like a Saturday. How good is that?

But the 30-Day Blitz is not just about exercise. It's a whole new way of life. Consider it like a cult – the Cult of Crosby! (Careful how you say that, as it might sound like you're talking about my lady parts.) This is about getting your mind into a place where you KNOW you can achieve what you want to achieve. I'm a firm believer that if your mind is on board and tells you that you're a winner then you will be. Your mind is a cunning character and can play all sorts of tricks on you when you're not watching. It can tell you you're ugly when you look in the mirror when really you're actually pretty fit. It can persuade you that you have a fat tummy when you really haven't. It can tell you that your hair smells because it needs a wash (although to be fair, your mind has a point – you stink of sheep) and it can be really mean and make you think you have a shit personality and nothing to offer the world. When we all know YOU ARE AMAZING.

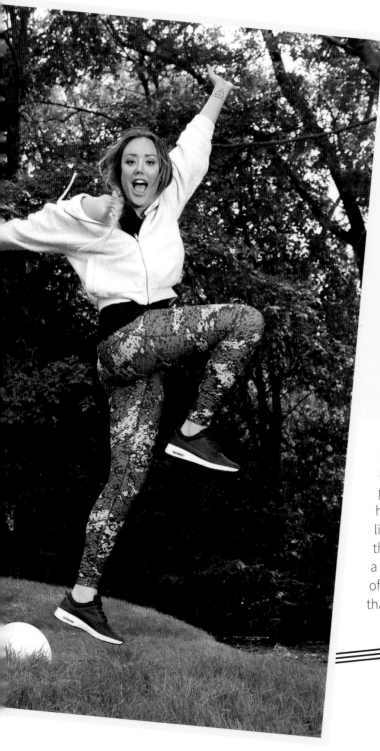

So, this is as much about training your mind as your body. And once your mind... actually, shall we give your mind a name? I feel a bit odd just saying 'mind'. Let's call it 'Mimi'! Yes, once Mimi is in the zone and on side then there will be nothing stopping you. Mimi is much more hardcore than your body. Mimi rules everything. So, this book will convince Mimi that this is all a brilliant idea and the best thing that will ever happen to you.

Now 30 days might seem like a long time but that's because Mimi is telling you it's a long time. If you put it into perspective and break down how long the average person lives (27,375 days apparently) then 30 days works out as just a measly 0.1095890410958904% of that (to be precise) – so take that measly Mimi!

CHARLOTTE'S WORDS OF WISDOM
EXERCISING WITH YOUR FRIENDS AND FAMILY

If you don't feel you can do my 30-Day Blitz on your own then you can always get a mate or your mam to do it with you for moral support.

As far as I'm concerned there are only ever positives to exercising with your mam. For a start you are always going to be better at all the workouts than she is. And it will always make you laugh which is also good for the endorphins – me mam Letitia's moves are a bit wooden so they always make me crack up laughing. Although she is a bit of a moaner when it comes to her shoulder – she's convinced she's hurt it somehow – so she uses that as an excuse not to do so much.

As far as exercising with friends goes, this has good and bad points. The good is that you will have company and someone to do it with and so you can catch up and gossip while you are exercising. The bad is that if one of your friends starts losing more weight than you it could do your head in.

But having them there as competition could also spur you on to do even better. Me and my mates got really competitive when we all got Fitbits – mine was a real motivator because I could challenge everyone… and then win! I was obsessed with beating every single person I knew.

GETTING STARTED

I know some people might look at me and think that I've got it all covered – that I have my body in check and already know what to do – but I still need the focus that something like a 30-Day Blitz can give you.

There are still times when I fall off the exercise wagon. Where do I start? When I'm working long hours, living out of a suitcase, birthdays… And then when I was rushed to hospital with an ectopic pregnancy and was out of action for weeks, I felt rubbish again because I couldn't look after myself or give myself that boost. And getting back into it afterwards was really tough too. Whatever your reason, don't give up, just get back on it.

Making friends with Exercise is always going to be hard in the beginning, but once you're even just a quarter of the way through the Blitz you will feel like you're starting to enjoy exercise more and more as you notice how much fitter you are.

This book is not going to force you to run a marathon in the first week. It's about starting from a place you are comfortable with and building up gently so you can actually stick it out and enjoy it.

A few years ago I couldn't even run up the stairs. The old me couldn't do a burpee at all. I couldn't run for the bus. When I used to get the train to London walking through the carriages to find a seat would get me down because I felt breathless.

I was physically embarrassed to walk into the gym – that's what would put me off! First of all, I didn't know what I was doing, and secondly, I didn't want people watching me sweating my arse off and looking hideous. But now I feel so confident that I can walk into any gym and know what I'm doing. Now I understand my body and know what works for me.

MY TRAINER IS YOUR TRAINER

David Souter, my trainer, has been with me from the very beginning of my fitness and weight loss journey. He met me back in 2013 when I was at my biggest and we went through the whole thing together: my first DVD (*3 Minute Belly Blitz*) and my second DVD (*3 Minute Bum Blitz*). That was a rollercoaster of an experience. In the end not only was he my trainer, he also felt like a family member – an uncle or an older brother. We still speak every single day. It's so amazing to have someone in my life who's so knowledgeable about fitness and is also a close friend who can give me boy advice.

I've learnt so much from David. I've learnt tips about how to train my body but I've also learnt not to stress about it. He wisely says, 'The second you start worrying about your weight is the second you start holding onto it.'

David has made me realise that for everything to work and for you to lose weight and get your body fine-tuned you need to be properly relaxed. He also told me that stress can affect your stomach – you can get bloated and feel constipated. If you're anxious about something or letting something get to you it stops your body doing what it needs to do. David has taught me to relax and to understand that weight comes off different people at different times – everyone is unique.

I asked David to use his magical powers on me and devise a workout plan that would burn fat, improve my fitness levels and also tone my whole body (I don't ask for much!). And by my body I also mean your body! I am used to most of his exercises but I made sure he included some beginner workouts as I like to train with my friends and wanted some easier options so they don't start moaning that they want to go to the pub halfway through! – which means you can choose which versions you do each time. David has also added some fun challenges at the end of each week to test my – and your! – fitness. The challenges really push me and make me burn even more fat! Go go go!

David is here helping you like he helps me – so think of him like your fairy godbrother!

EXERCISE THAT DOESN'T FEEL LIKE EXERCISE

In the Blitz I've suggested some fun extra activities to do on a Sunday that have the added benefit of helping with your fitness. If you don't fancy my suggestions, here are some others you can try instead.

1. Dancing
In a nightclub or in your kitchen.

2. Housework
Once I had to mop the whole kitchen and sitting room and I was so knackered afterwards!

3. Sex
Instead of H.I.T. circuits try some H.I.F. – High Intensity F***ing.

4. Weight lifting
I use my dogs or you could ask a friend to lend you their baby.

5. TV sit-ups
I don't even bother getting on the floor; I just do them on the sofa.

6. Stair runs
Just pretend you've left your straighteners on and are worried your favourite jacket will catch fire – that will make you sprint right up them!

7. Hoovering
Just make sure you lunge when you're pushing the Hoover. And if you've got a lawn to mow, lunge when you're pushing the mower too. Not too wide mind, you don't want to get your foot caught in the blade – then you won't be able to do any exercise at all and you'll be suing me for ruining your life because you can't walk.

8. Morning planks
Make getting out of bed exciting by rolling out and going straight into a plank.

9. Fridge squats
You can squat literally every time you look in the fridge for something to eat.

10. Waving at the neighbours
Lift your arms up and down in a diagonal motion. They will think you're really lovely and friendly and you'll get rid of your bingo wings at the same time.

FOOD FOR THOUGHT

(AND I MEAN THAT BECAUSE IT'S GOOD
FOR YOUR BRAIN WHEN YOU EAT BETTER!)

Not only has my attitude to exercise changed, but the way I look at food is so different now too. As soon as I started learning about what to eat and cook my eating habits completely changed. Nowadays I'm always very conscious that I need to be eating good, healthy food. That's what my 30-Day Blitz is all about. Eating good, healthy food in moderation. All the meals in this book have been carefully planned and calorie counted to ensure they are nutritionally balanced. The recipes are packed with lean protein, good-for-you fats and slow-release carbs, which means they won't leave you raging for an iced doughnut! This is a diet to stick to over 30 days when you want a kick-start.

There have been some really bad diets and plans that people have followed in the past. Back in the 1960s there was one called the 'wine and eggs diet' which told you to drink a glass of wine for breakfast and lunch and half a bottle for dinner! Plus a load of eggs. Can you even believe it?! If you did that you would just be drunk and farting the whole time. There's another called the 'Master Cleanse' that Beyoncé was rumoured to have done before she was in *Dreamgirls*. It involves drinking something like syrup, lemon and cayenne pepper – all great if you want to be miserable the whole time and have no mates because of your bad breath. DO NOT TRY THESE!

Holly Hagan and I once tried the 'baby food diet' – where you eat baby food the whole time – for three days. It was ridiculous because we looked so stupid sitting with our tiny pots of mashed-up peas at the dinner table. And we were just starving the whole time.

Someone once told me that if you want to eat less you should put your meal on a blue plate... because apparently the colour blue puts you off food!

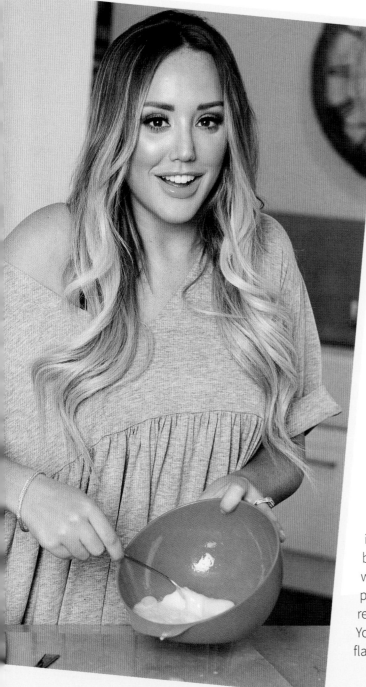

I can actually imagine that working a little bit because the thought of eating off a blue plate is making me feel a bit ill.

I'm trying to eat less red meat for lots of reasons and I definitely don't eat it on a date because I will end up asleep at the table in a food coma! The recipes in this book are much more fish- and veg-based than heavy meats – and you can get loads of great protein from things like eggs without having to eat meat.

This book is designed for people who live and work and don't have time to make huge meals every day. I know you need to have something that fits in with your life. You just need to prepare a bit the night before, or at the weekend if that's easier. But it honestly won't be a pain. It will be easy. By making an extra effort with prep you'll be cutting back on processed foods, which means less refined sugars, bad fats and salt. You'll improve your digestion, get a flat belly and banish bloating.

I know I've always talked about the brilliant thing about having a cheat day on my diet plans before… but the 30-Day Blitz is a bit more demanding. However, the commitment will be worth it, I promise! So, no alcohol for a start! And instead of cheat days we've included some sweet treats and snacks to keep you going. Or instead I like to have a rice cake, two small squares of dark chocolate or a Yobu frozen yoghurt lolly, which are unreal.

But IF (and I mean IIIIIFFF) you do end up falling off the food wagon I don't want you to stop and not look at the book again. I don't want this book being used as a doorstop or a handy little stabiliser for the wonky leg on your kitchen table. I want this book to be your bible. So, if you feel like you've failed on one meal or accidentally eaten a packet of crisps (what did they do, just fly into your mouth?) don't tell anyone, just turn the page and keep going.

YOU ARE WHAT YOU POO

I used to be constantly getting bloated and had really bad bowels – I found it difficult to go to the toilet and poo. I thought it was just boys who went for regular poos every day, but then I spoke to a few of my friends like Sophie who told me very matter-of-factly that she has daily poos! It was then I realised there was something wrong with me because sometimes I would go for four days without a poo and my stomach would be rock solid. By keeping a diary I discovered I might be intolerant to some common ingredients so I cut them out – my stomach went flatter and I pooed and pooed! It was the best thing I have ever done. Pooing has changed my life!

Why not keep a diary to see the effect the food plan has on your body? Different foods can affect people in different ways – keeping a diary can help you narrow down the foods that affect you. And poo can be a great indicator of the overall health of your system.

CHARLOTTE'S WORDS OF WISDOM

GET A COMPLIMENTS BLITZ

Sometimes it's good to get a compliments blitz to spur you on. Today I asked me mam and my mate Sophie to send me a list of five good things about me and this is what they wrote. (Sophie wins over Mam by the way!) It brought a tear to my eye when I read those comments. I need to start talking to myself in the mirror a bit more and giving myself some of that unconditional love (and great advice!).
Give it a go!

Mam:
1. You have the best legs I have ever seen.
2. You have a very kind and pure heart.
3. You have a very funny, dry sense of humour.
4. You will always do anything for your brother and look after him when I'm away.
5. You have an amazing work ethic and give 100% to everything you do.

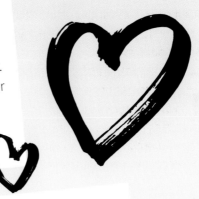

Sophie:
1. You brighten up every single room you walk into.
2. People underestimate you – you're one of the most business-minded and successful people I know.
3. You are extremely generous and loving.
4. You're great at giving advice (but bad at taking it).
5. When you love someone, you love them unconditionally.

CHARLOTTE'S RULES FOR SUCCESS

Before you start on the 30-Day Blitz I want you to read these rules. Together they're my mantra to guide you through the next 30 days and beyond:

1. Work hard

Even if you haven't had a break, even if you're working till late, never ever let it get you down. Because if you're working hard it means that you are miles ahead of anyone else who is just sitting at home having a day off. There have been times when I've been working non-stop until two or three in the morning and felt tired and sick. But I tell myself that I'm really lucky to have been asked to do these shows, and I should feel GREAT. The same attitude carried me through my bar shift when I used to work at Ttonic in Sunderland and through the long hours on the phone at a call centre.

2. Always make something your own

Have your own ideas and put your own spin on something. The last thing people want to see is something that 500 other people have done before – so don't be boring.

3. Wake up in the morning and say out loud three things you are thankful for

Not only will this help you start the day feeling grateful, lucky and extremely positive, it will automatically rid you of anything negative. We all have three things to be happy about and I feel so lucky with my life. This morning I woke up and said:

Thank you for my good health.
Thank you for my many amazing work opportunities.
Thank you for my loving and amazing friends and family.

4. Be professional in everything you do

Even if you're a bit crazy at times or feel moody still try to be professional. Be kind to everyone around you. Put in 110% and get the job done.

5. Don't be afraid to fail

This is one I struggle to stick to. I worry and stress a lot that the things I'm working on won't do well – that people may not want to watch my shows or won't like something I've brought out. When really I should think, 'Why on earth does it matter?' All that matters is that you gave it a go and you achieved something. It's your failures that are the greatest lessons you grow and learn from – so be grateful for the things that sometimes don't go so well.

6. Get a dog

Dogs are a man's – or a WOMAN'S – best friend. They bring so many joys in life. A walk a day with your dog gets the air into your lungs, and is great for the heart and the mind. I feel my dogs have helped me succeed in life. Thanks Rhubarb and Baby (and now Banana too)!

7. Your parents aren't always right

(Even though sometimes they are.) If I'd listened to me mam then I wouldn't have gone into *Geordie Shore* and none of my crazy life since then would have happened. And that would've been BORINGGGG. Don't do something because it's what your parents want of you. Always do it for you.

8. Walk around the house naked

Not only does it make you feel empowered, it's always good to appreciate where it all started! Rolling naked from the womb!

9. Fart out loud

Imagine it's the negative vibes passing out of your body and just let them go! There's never anything good about keeping a fart in! No matter where you are or who you're with – release it, guys.

10. Be nice to strangers

Ask people how their day was or tell them, 'You've got nice hair!' I was in a spa once and an American man getting some water started speaking to me. Instead of avoiding him I said, 'I love the accent, where are you from?' We had a chat and it felt really nice to be interested in another human being!

HOW TO FOLLOW THE 30-DAY BLITZ

So here we go! I promise that if you follow my plan for the full 30 days you will not only feel UHMAZING but you will also look like a new person (by that I mean a much fitter and healthier one, not that you will have a face transplant and suddenly look like one of your neighbours). You'll see a difference in how your clothes fit. You will want a whole new wardrobe to show off your new body and you will not be able to stop admiring yourself in the mirror! That's not all. Without realising, by following this plan you will end up learning loads of healthy eating principles which, once you've got them in your brain, will keep you on the right track well after the 30 days. We've designed the plan to deliver the balance of nutrients you need for beautiful looking skin, luscious hair and nails as well as more energy than you have ever had in your life. You will power through the workouts and challenges as if you're a superhero.

It's OK to swap days or repeat them but don't be tempted to swap individual meals as each day is calculated to ensure you get a mix of all the food groups and nutrients you need to smash my training programme! If there's one ingredient that really makes you feel sick and you're thinking, 'Why, Charlotte? Why? I can't eat that!' then you can exchange it for something that does the same job, like trout for salmon or watercress for spinach.

I try to drink three litres of low-calorie fluid every day – usually water, I bloody love drinking water, especially when I'm training. To remind you to drink plenty of fluids, I've added pictures of eight glasses to the plan for each day. (And while I was at it, I added a reminder to get some sleep too.)

I've based my menu plan on two people sharing but to save time and effort some of the recipes make portions to store or freeze so you don't have to think about cooking every day (you do have a life after all!). The plan takes account of these which means there's minimal wastage plus you'll have a few extra portions to keep the healthy eating going once you've finished the 30 days.

At the weekend I always want to get a few mates round so I've included a couple of party meals to enjoy with your friends.

Each day of the plan gives you around 1500 calories, which allows room for an energising or protein-packed snack to help you recover after exercise, some milk or plant-based equivalent (I like almond milk) for adding to hot drinks and even the odd sweet 'treat' for that occasion when you just need a little something. Including these extras will help you stick to the plan and give you the fuel you need to exercise to your max.

The plan also gives you at least five of your 'five a day' and keeps within the daily recommended quantities of fat, saturated fats, sugar and salt. A balanced diet should also include two portions of fish or seafood each week, one of these should be an oily one like salmon, fresh tuna, trout or mackerel.

I am always running about like a loon and with such a hectic lifestyle I often have to grab and go – my 30-Day Blitz has to work for me and you so you'll find breakfasts that you can stash in your bag, like my yummy Sweet Potato Muffins, and lunches that can be packed up and taken to work.

Now I'm trying to eat less meat, and especially red meat, I've kept recipes that include it to a minimum, but I've not cut them out completely. That's because lean meat is a great source of protein, which helps tone and shape your muscles and it's a brilliant source of energising iron. Where relevant in the plan I've provided a veggie option, so if you don't eat meat I haven't forgotten you! On each of the meat recipes you'll find alternatives to make it veggie. Just remember, though, it's the plan that has been calorie counted and nutrient checked so changing to veggie ingredients might alter it slightly.

I've tried to include lots of variety, we can all get stuck in a food rut, eating the same things day after day. For those doing the Blitz along with me, look out for shopping lists and other tips on my social media accounts. Blitz time can be a good time to try something new. So, bring it on. Let's get blitzing!

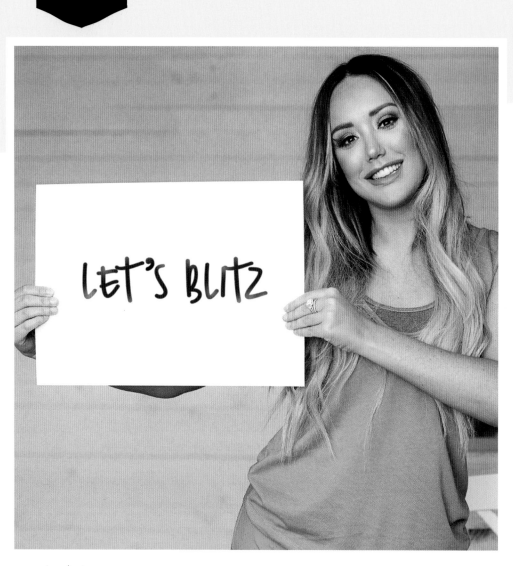

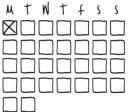

OK, it's Day 1 my friends! This is the day to say goodbye to all those bad habits and shoo them out of your bedroom door like a bad smell. This is the start of the journey. And it's going to be fun! If this is the first time you've moved from the sofa in weeks the exercises below are the intermediate level, but if you turn to the pages, you can see some easier beginners' alternatives. So don't panic! Throughout the plan we'll be putting things in the fridge and freezer to use later on – today you'll have leftovers of everything to save for another day.

MENU

Breakfast:

All-in-One Baked Egg Cups
(see p96)

Lunch:

Sweet Potato, Lentil & Spinach Soup *(see p127)*

Dinner:

Vegetable Lasagne
(see p152)

Plus:

Hummus
(see p180–1)

WORKOUT

💗 **Warm-Up** *(see pp190–3)*

Do 25 seconds each of the following:

– Spidy Step & Reach *(see pp194–5)*
– Skywalkers *(see pp196–7)*
– Cowgirl Burpees *(see pp198–9)*
– Box Knee & Kick Out *(see pp200–1)*
– Star Jump & Front Kick *(see pp202–3)*
– Crunch & Alt Knee *(see pp204–5)*

🌀 **Repeat the whole workout**

🏃 **Stretches & Cool-Down** *(see pp214–7)*

GLASSES of WATER

HOURS of SLEEP

| PM | | | | | AM | | | | | | | | | | | | | | | | PM | | | |
| 7 | 8 | 9 | 10 | 11 | 12 | 1 | 2 | 3 | 4 | 5 | 6 | 7 | 8 | 9 | 10 | 11 | 12 | 1 | 2 | 3 | 4 |

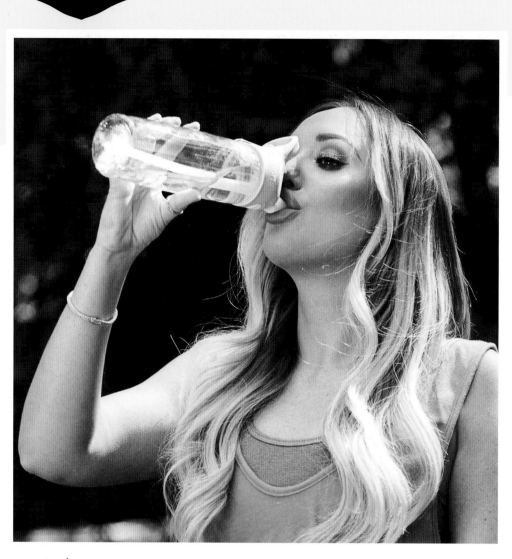

M T W T F S S

☒ ☒ ☐ ☐ ☐ ☐ ☐
☐ ☐ ☐ ☐ ☐ ☐ ☐
☐ ☐ ☐ ☐ ☐ ☐ ☐
☐ ☐ ☐ ☐ ☐ ☐ ☐
☐ ☐

I cannot stress enough how important it is to have water! The more you drink, the better your skin, your digestion and your inner body movements (I mean pooing). Water gets your whole system flushed out to perfection! When I was younger I always used to love juice or fizzy drinks but now my love affair is with the clear stuff from the tap. It's all about the H2O if you want to be in the know! (And it's better for your teeth too.) Make sure you colour in the chart so you know what you are drinking and never forget to have enough. Usually two litres or eight glasses is recommended although I always try to drink three litres a day. I am a watering machine!

MENU

Breakfast:

All-in-One Baked Egg Cups
(leftover from Day 1)

Lunch:

Vegetable Lasagne
(leftover from Day 1)

Dinner:

Courgetti with Spicy
Cashew Pesto *(see p158)*

Plus:

Hummus *(see pp180–1)*

WORKOUT

💜 **Warm-Up** *(see pp190–3)*

Do 25 seconds each of the following:

– Spidy Step & Reach *(see pp194–5)*
– Skywalkers *(see pp196–7)*
– Cowgirl Burpees *(see pp198–9)*
– Box Knee & Kick Out *(see pp200–1)*
– Star Jump & Front Kick *(see pp202–3)*
– Crunch & Alt Knee *(see pp204–5)*

🔄 **Repeat the whole workout**

🤸 **Stretches & Cool-Down** *(see pp214–7)*

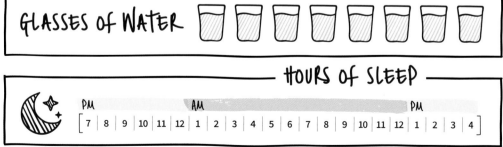

GLASSES of WATER

HOURS of SLEEP

PM · AM · PM

[7 | 8 | 9 | 10 | 11 | 12 | 1 | 2 | 3 | 4 | 5 | 6 | 7 | 8 | 9 | 10 | 11 | 12 | 1 | 2 | 3 | 4]

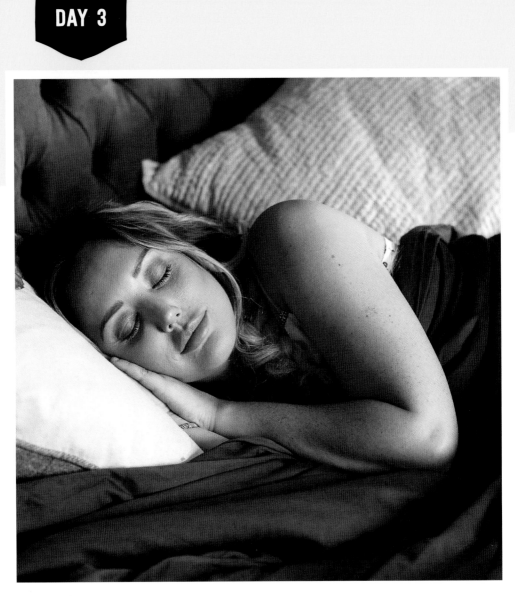

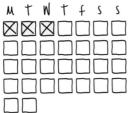

Get lots of sleep. I might sound like your mam, but sleep is good for you! The best thing to get you looking and feeling your best (apart from water like I told you yesterday) is sleep. Try to get at least seven hours every night. And you're not going to have a really restful night if your room is like a bombsite. So you will need to face up to it and blitz your bedroom. Get everything in order. I have underwear all over the place – clean and dirty – so that's the first thing I need to sort out.

MENU

Breakfast:

Herby Falafel Waffles with Poached Eggs *(see pp92–3)*

Lunch:

Courgetti with Spicy Cashew Pesto
(leftover from Day 2)

Dinner:

Garlic Chilli Prawns with Wild Rice & Green Beans
(see p161)

Plus:

Hummus *(see pp180–1)*

WORKOUT

💗 **Warm-Up** *(see pp190–3)*

Do 25 seconds each of the following:

– Spidy Step & Reach *(see pp194–5)*
– Skywalkers *(see pp196–7)*
– Cowgirl Burpees *(see pp198–9)*
– Box Knee & Kick Out *(see pp200–1)*
– Star Jump & Front Kick *(see pp202–3)*
– Crunch & Alt Knee *(see pp204–5)*

🔄 **Repeat the whole workout**

🧘 **Stretches & Cool-Down** *(see pp214–7)*

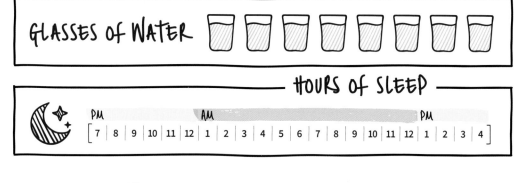

GLASSES of WATER

HOURS of SLEEP

PM | AM | PM
[7 | 8 | 9 | 10 | 11 | 12 | 1 | 2 | 3 | 4 | 5 | 6 | 7 | 8 | 9 | 10 | 11 | 12 | 1 | 2 | 3 | 4]

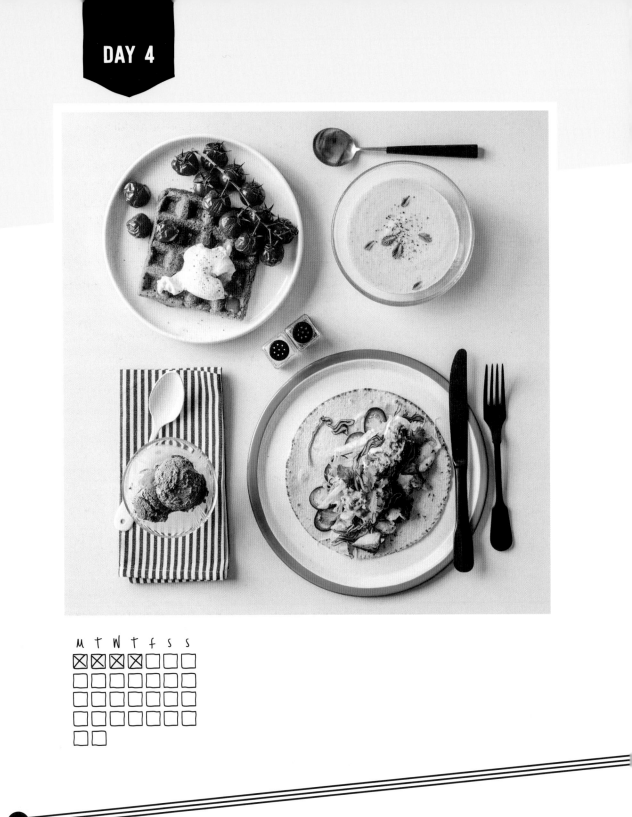

See how pretty this meal plan looks! These waffles are almost too beautiful to put in your stomach for breakfast – they should be on the wall. (That's a joke by the way, I don't want you turning waffles into wallpaper.) But I seriously believe that if you make an effort to get your food looking nice on a plate it makes you enjoy it more. It shows you care about what you're putting inside. And as for your outside – how cool is the name cowgirl burpees? I love how David gives funny names for things. Don't mess with him or his workouts. They are the business.

MENU

Breakfast:

Herby Falafel Waffles with Poached Eggs *(use leftover waffles from Day 3, see pp92–3 for the eggs)*

Lunch:

Cucumber & Mint Soup *(see p122)*

Dinner:

Cod Tacos with Crème Frâiche & Guacamole *(see p144)*

Plus:

Berry Frozen Yoghurt *(see p170)*

WORKOUT

💜 **Warm-Up** *(see pp190–3)*

Do 25 seconds each of the following:

– Spidy Step & Reach *(see pp194–5)*
– Skywalkers *(see pp196–7)*
– Cowgirl Burpees *(see pp198–9)*
– Box Knee & Kick Out *(see pp200–1)*
– Star Jump & Front Kick *(see pp202–3)*
– Crunch & Alt Knee *(see pp204–5)*

🌀 **Repeat the workout two more times**

🐾 **Stretches & Cool-Down** *(see pp214–7)*

GLASSES of WATER

HOURS of SLEEP

PM					AM												PM			
7	8	9	10	11	12	1	2	3	4	5	6	7	8	9	10	11	12	1	2	3	4

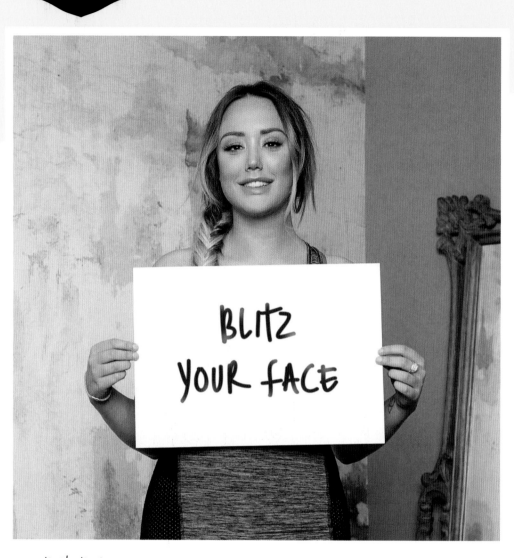

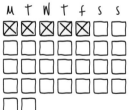

You're at the end of the week already – hurrah! As it's Friday night you deserve a bit of pampering before the weekend. Think of it as my treat to you! Blitz your face. Put on a face pack, pluck and dye your eyebrows, do a blackhead peel in the bath and give your chin a massage (apparently this can stop you getting a double chin). This is where you look at yourself in the mirror and wave the old tired, sluggish creature in front of you goodbye! Soon she will be replaced by a bright sparkly-eyed being who can't stop smiling. She will also have good hair.

MENU

Breakfast:

Green Smoothie with Greek Yoghurt *(see p90)*

Lunch:

Rainbow Noodles with Sweet & Spicy Sauce *(see p110)*

Dinner:

Turkey Chilli con Carne with Shredded Green Veg *(see p156)*

Plus:

Guacamole & veg sticks *(see p182)*

WORKOUT

💗 **Warm-Up** *(see pp190–3)*

Do 25 seconds each of the following:

– Spidy Step & Reach *(see pp194–5)*
– Skywalkers *(see pp196–7)*
– Cowgirl Burpees *(see pp198–9)*
– Box Knee & Kick Out *(see pp200–1)*
– Star Jump & Front Kick *(see pp202–3)*
– Crunch & Alt Knee *(see pp204–5)*

🔄 **Repeat the workout two more times**

🤸 **Stretches & Cool-Down** *(see pp214–7)*

GLASSES of WATER

HOURS of SLEEP

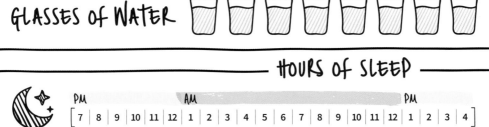

PM					AM											PM			
7	8	9	10	11	12	1	2	3	4	5	6	7	8	9	10	11	12	1	2	3	4

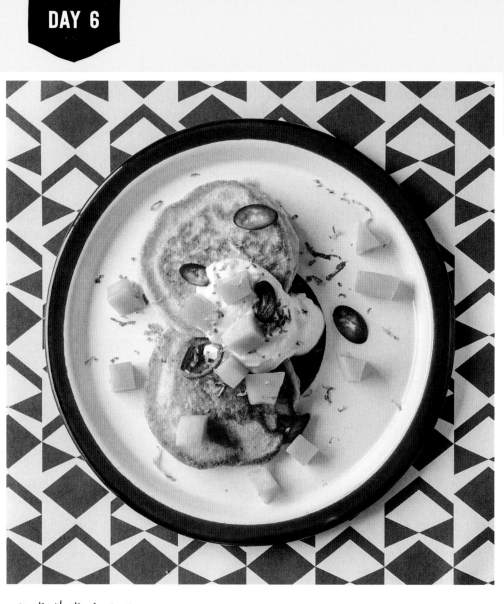

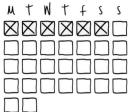

It's the weekend so I've decided to treat you with a picture of PANCAKES! And the beauty of these pancakes is that they are actually healthy for you. My bum used to be like a pancake but it was never as tasty as this one. And thinking about tasty bums, it's time to shake things up with the first of our Saturday challenges – this is instead of the workout so you don't burn out. You can switch between mountain climbers and plank as many times as you want, but stop the clock as soon as you can't do any more and aim to beat your results each round.

MENU

Breakfast:

Coconut Pancakes with Mango & Lime Yoghurt
(see p98)

Lunch:

Sweet Potato, Lentil & Spinach Soup
(defrosted from Day 1)

Dinner:

Tuna, Bean & Rough Romesco Salad
(see p150)

Plus:

Berry Frozen Yoghurt
(stored in the freezer from Day 4)

WORKOUT

⭐ SATURDAY CHALLENGE ⭐

💗 **Warm-Up** *(see pp190–3)*

For as long as you can:

– Mountain Climbers *(see pp206–7)*
  into Plank *(see p197)*

🌀 **Rest, then repeat the challenge two more times**

〰️ **Stretches & Cool-Down** *(see pp214–7)*

GLASSES OF WATER

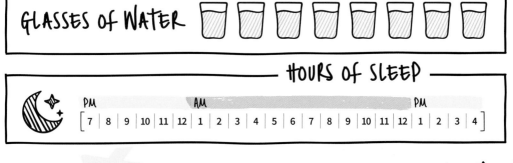

HOURS OF SLEEP

PM | AM | PM

[7 | 8 | 9 | 10 | 11 | 12 | 1 | 2 | 3 | 4 | 5 | 6 | 7 | 8 | 9 | 10 | 11 | 12 | 1 | 2 | 3 | 4]

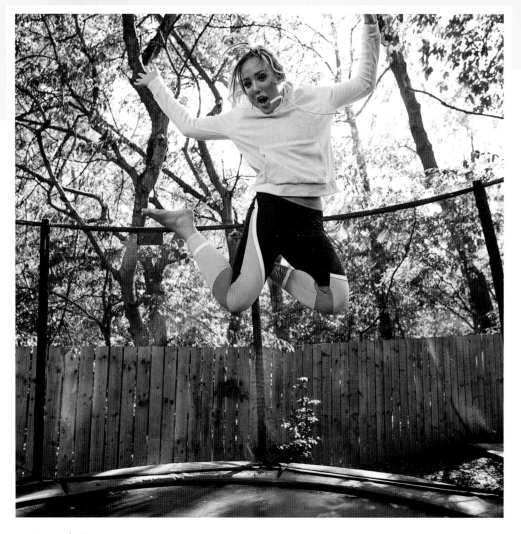

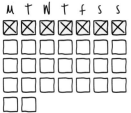

Sundays are just about fun activities that are also keeping you fit – you need a rest day (plus I don't want to scare you off in the first week!). So today I've decided you should go trampolining! I bought this trampoline for my brother Nathaniel but I use it more than he does. If you don't have one of your own you could go to a trampoline park. It's really fun, especially because people always look ridiculous on trampolines so it makes you laugh. And as it's Sunday treat yourself to a roast. I love a roast (so does me mam Letitia but she always manages to cock it up somehow). And by making a roast chicken at the weekend you have the basis for the next two days' lunches. Clever huh?

MENU

Breakfast:
Breakfast Tray Bake *(see p95)*

Lunch:
All Green Soup *(see p114)*

Dinner:
Roast Chicken, Roast Veg &
Steamed Greens *(see pp164–5)*

Plus:
Poached Pears with
Vanilla Yoghurt *(see p172)*

WORKOUT

30 MINUTES' TRAMPOLINING*

*Or any extra exercise *(see p13)*

GLASSES OF WATER

HOURS OF SLEEP

PM | AM | PM

[7 | 8 | 9 | 10 | 11 | 12 | 1 | 2 | 3 | 4 | 5 | 6 | 7 | 8 | 9 | 10 | 11 | 12 | 1 | 2 | 3 | 4]

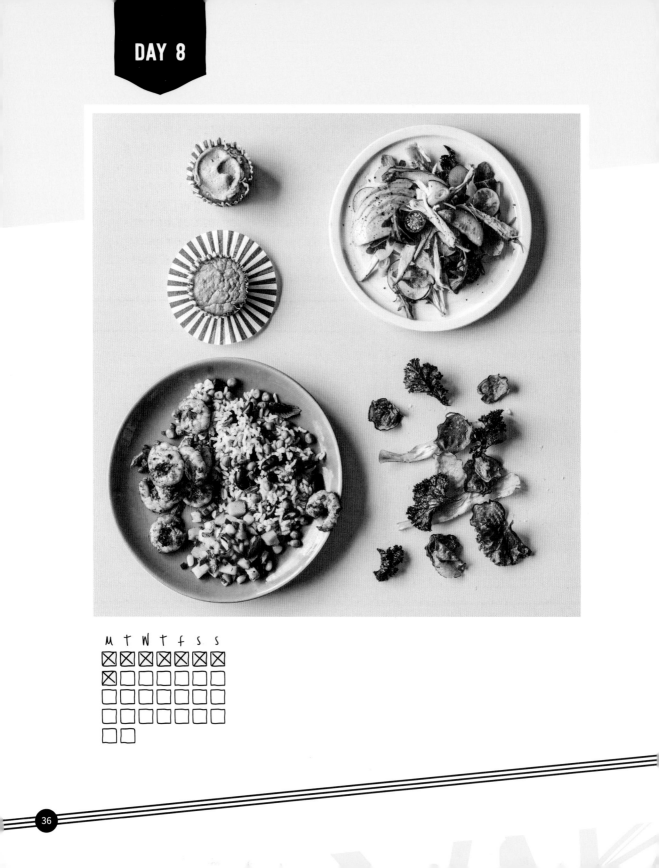

I've added a new exercise and reversed the order to keep it interesting. I've also increased the amount of time (sorry… but what did you think this was, a holiday?!). All that extra exercise deserves muffins and crisps! Make sure you're not tempted to eat them all though – put them in an airtight container (not together) for later in the week. Start the week by blitzing your fridge. Chuck out everything bad for you then give the whole thing a good clean. When was the last time you cared about that poor fridge? This is now the most important vessel in your life… so you need to give it the same TLC as you give your hair. Wash it, brush it, stroke it. The fridge is your friend.

MENU

Breakfast:

Sweet Potato Muffins
(see p102)

Lunch:

Roast Chicken Salad *(see p116)*

Dinner:

Jerk Prawns, Rice & Peas with Mango, Pineapple & Chilli Salsa *(see p134)*

Plus:

Vegetable Crisps *(see p178)*

WORKOUT

Warm-Up *(see pp190–3)*

Do 30 seconds each of the following:

– Crunch & Alt Knee *(see pp204–5)*
– Star Jump & Front Kick *(see pp202–3)*
– Box Knee & Kick Out *(see pp200–1)*
– Cowgirl Burpees *(see pp198–9)*
– Skywalkers *(see pp196–7)*
– Spidy Step & Reach *(see pp194–5)*
– Lateral Jabs & Jacks *(see pp208–9)*

Repeat the whole workout

Stretches & Cool-Down *(see pp214–7)*

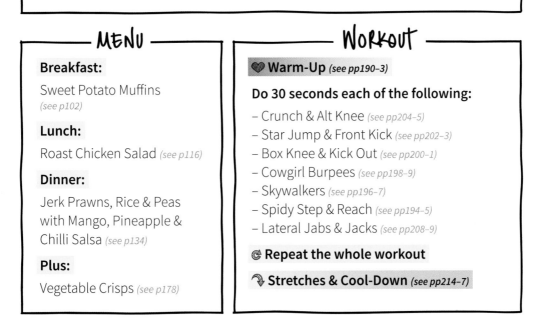

GLASSES OF WATER

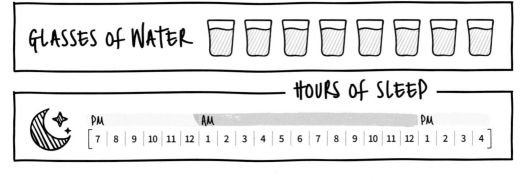

HOURS OF SLEEP

PM · AM · PM

[7 | 8 | 9 | 10 | 11 | 12 | 1 | 2 | 3 | 4 | 5 | 6 | 7 | 8 | 9 | 10 | 11 | 12 | 1 | 2 | 3 | 4]

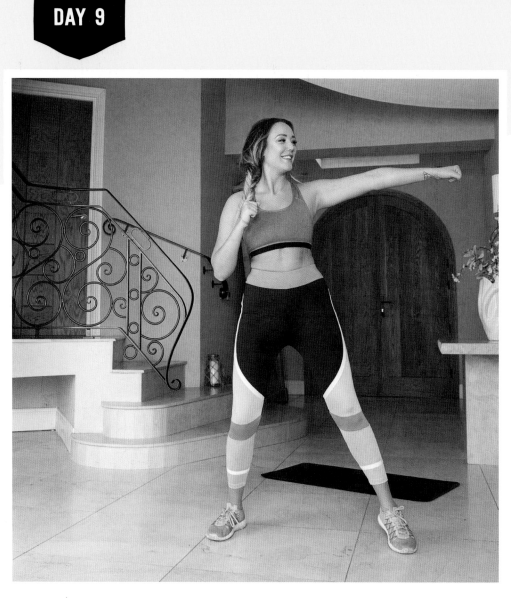

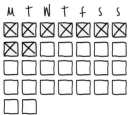

If you haven't put the right fuel into your body and you haven't had enough sleep then you're not going to work out to the best of your ability. Think of yourself as a mechanic fine-tuning a brilliant racing car. You need to be able to go vroom on the track and leave everything else for dust! When you're exercising you always use loads of energy so if you do the workout before breakfast you'll really benefit from the carbs and proteins in the smoothie.

MENU

Breakfast:

Almond & Berry Smoothie *(see p104)*

Lunch:

Bang Bang Chicken Lettuce Wraps *(see p124)*

Dinner:

Cottage Pie with Root Veg Mash *(see p160)*

Plus:

Vegetable Crisps *(stored from Day 8)*

WORKOUT

🫀 **Warm-Up** *(see pp190–3)*

Do 30 seconds each of the following:

– Crunch & Alt Knee *(see pp204–5)*
– Star Jump & Front Kick *(see pp202–3)*
– Box Knee & Kick Out *(see pp200–1)*
– Cowgirl Burpees *(see pp198–9)*
– Skywalkers *(see pp196–7)*
– Spidy Step & Reach *(see pp194–5)*
– Lateral Jabs & Jacks *(see pp208–9)*

🔄 **Repeat the whole workout**

🧘 **Stretches & Cool-Down** *(see pp214–7)*

GLASSES of WATER

HOURS of SLEEP

PM					AM											PM			
7	8	9	10	11	12	1	2	3	4	5	6	7	8	9	10	11	12	1	2	3	4

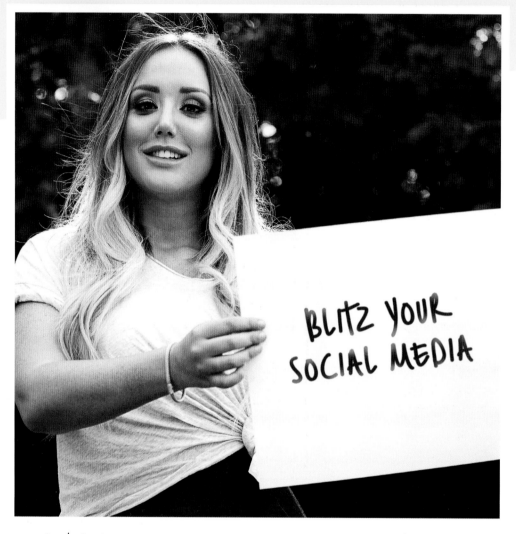

BLITZ YOUR SOCIAL MEDIA

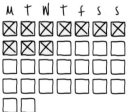

Watch out chocoholics, these Chocolate Bombs are very yummy. Keep them as a treat for when you've completed your workout (they are NOT to be consumed all in one session!). While you're eating them why not blitz your social media? Get rid of the trolls and the people whose Instagram accounts are boring or making you jealous. There is no need to have anyone on your feed that doesn't make you feel good. Instagram is a place for joy and niceness – you don't need negativity. Block anyone who is really annoying you. That's what the blocking mechanism is for!

MENU

Breakfast:

Sweet Potato Muffins
(see p102)

Lunch:

All Green Soup
(defrosted from Day 7)

Dinner:

Roasted Salmon with Slaw in Citrus Dressing *(see p136)*

Plus:

Chocolate Bombs *(see p173)*

WORKOUT

🩵 **Warm-Up** *(see pp190–3)*

Do 30 seconds each of the following:

– Crunch & Alt Knee *(see pp204–5)*
– Star Jump & Front Kick *(see pp202–3)*
– Box Knee & Kick Out *(see pp200–1)*
– Cowgirl Burpees *(see pp198–9)*
– Skywalkers *(see pp196–7)*
– Spidy Step & Reach *(see pp194–5)*
– Lateral Jabs & Jacks *(see pp208–9)*

🔄 **Repeat the whole workout**

🐾 **Stretches & Cool-Down** *(see pp214–7)*

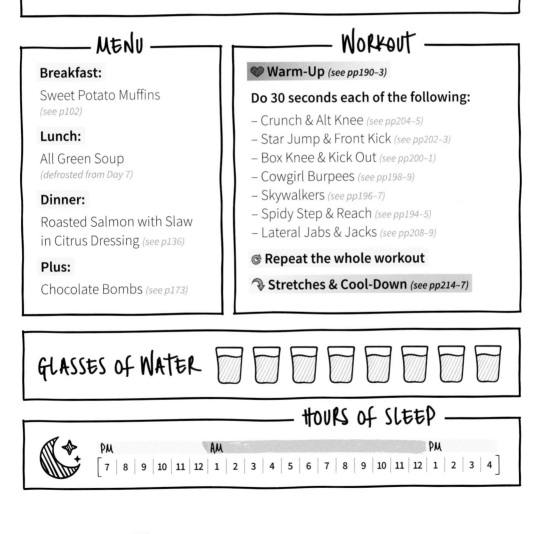

GLASSES OF WATER

HOURS OF SLEEP

PM					AM												PM			
7	8	9	10	11	12	1	2	3	4	5	6	7	8	9	10	11	12	1	2	3	4

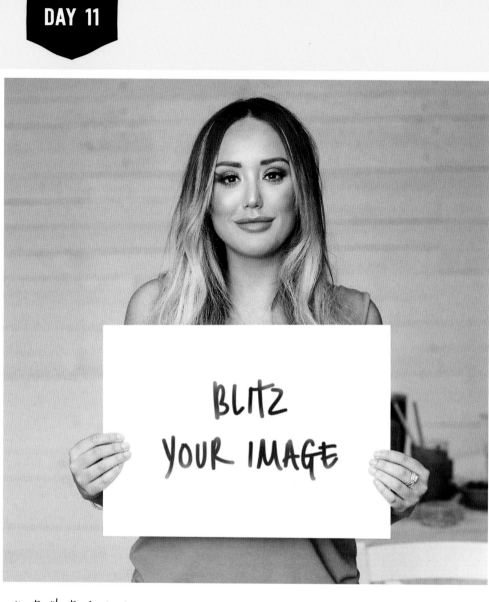

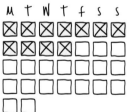

This is about blitzing your old image and building up a spanking new one that you won't even recognise in a few days time. Get rid of all those bad memories of the old version of you. Remember that girl who had a spot last month? *See ya spot face*! And how about that time you looked in the mirror and thought 'look at those bags under your eyes'? *Bye bye bag lady*! These exercises will give you loads of energy and get you in the mood for food (which you can only eat when you've done my exercises below!).

MENU

Breakfast:
Overnight Peanut Butter Oats with Apple Slices
(see p91)

Lunch:
Roasted Salmon with Slaw in Citrus Dressing
(leftover from Day 10)

Lunch:
Vegetable Lasagne
(defrosted from Day 1)

Plus:
Vegetable Crisps *(see p178)*

WORKOUT

💜 **Warm-Up** *(see pp190–3)*

Do 30 seconds each of the following:
– Crunch & Alt Knee *(see pp204–5)*
– Star Jump & Front Kick *(see pp202–3)*
– Box Knee & Kick Out *(see pp200–1)*
– Cowgirl Burpees *(see pp198–9)*
– Skywalkers *(see pp196–7)*
– Spidy Step & Reach *(see pp194–5)*
– Lateral Jabs & Jacks *(see pp208–9)*

🔄 **Repeat the workout two more times**

🌿 **Stretches & Cool-Down** *(see pp214–7)*

GLASSES of WATER

HOURS of SLEEP

PM   AM   PM

[7 | 8 | 9 | 10 | 11 | 12 | 1 | 2 | 3 | 4 | 5 | 6 | 7 | 8 | 9 | 10 | 11 | 12 | 1 | 2 | 3 | 4]

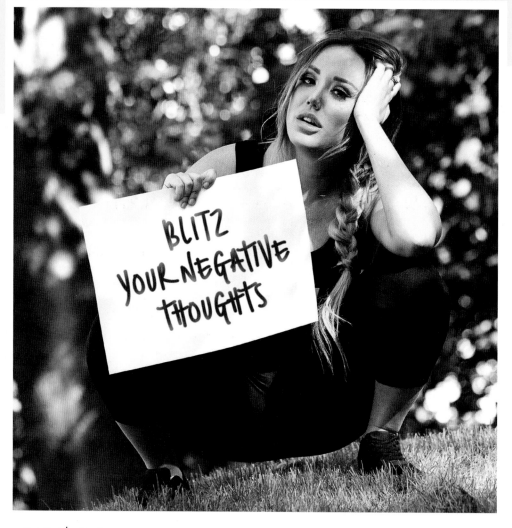

BLITZ YOUR NEGATIVE THOUGHTS

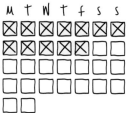

M T W T F S S

Blitz your negative thoughts. Write all your worst thoughts on a piece of paper and think about how ridiculous they are. Then cross them off and tell yourself they mean nothing. I get really bad death anxiety and lie in bed thinking about dying and the emptiness of it being all over. I literally think about death every day. I need to remind myself this is not going to happen for years and years and focus on the great exciting things I have ahead of me. So, whatever your bad thoughts are, write them down and blitz them out of your mind! And get ready for the weekend.

MENU

Breakfast:

Sweet Potato Muffins *(see p102)*

Lunch:

Red Lentil, Pepper & Chorizo Soup *(see p126)*

Dinner:

Crispy Coconut Cod with Pineapple Rice *(see p157)*

Plus:

Chocolate Bombs *(stored from Day 10)*

WORKOUT

💗 **Warm-Up** *(see pp190–3)*

Do 30 seconds each of the following:

– Crunch & Alt Knee *(see pp204–5)*
– Star Jump & Front Kick *(see pp202–3)*
– Box Knee & Kick Out *(see pp200–1)*
– Cowgirl Burpees *(see pp198–9)*
– Skywalkers *(see pp196–7)*
– Spidy Step & Reach *(see pp194–5)*
– Lateral Jabs & Jacks *(see pp208–9)*

🌀 **Repeat the workout two more times**

🔽 **Stretches & Cool-Down** *(see pp214–7)*

GLASSES OF WATER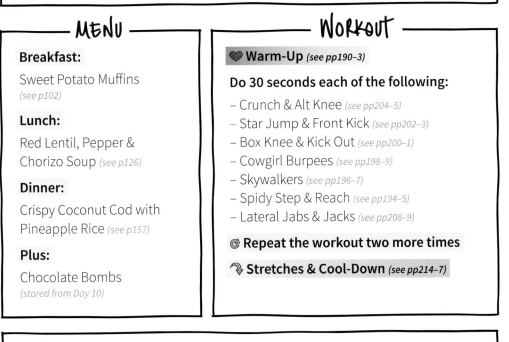

HOURS OF SLEEP

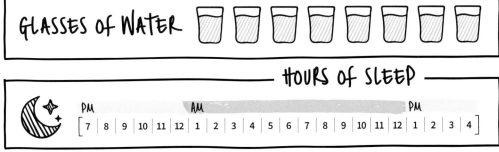

PM					AM											PM			
7	8	9	10	11	12	1	2	3	4	5	6	7	8	9	10	11	12	1	2	3	4

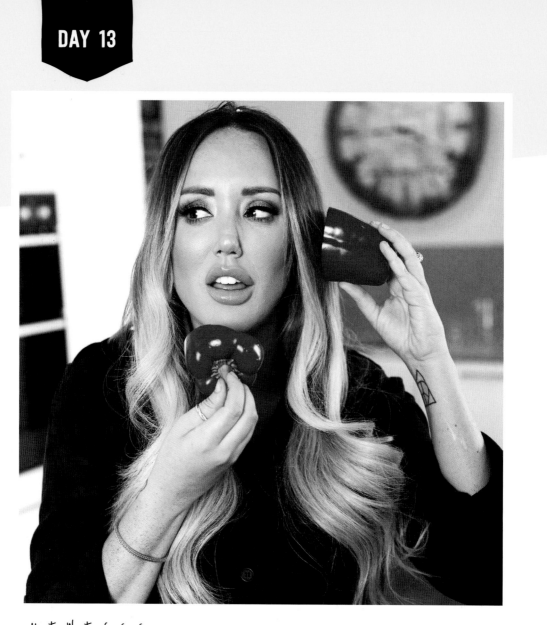

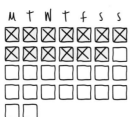

You've got more time on your hands at the weekend so it's OK for these recipes to take a bit longer. I love making sure my kitchen is all nicely lit and I have the radio on and dance and sing to myself while I'm preparing the food (just don't use a knife as a microphone… a whisk is much safer). This Saturday challenge is about you really pushing yourself to do repeats of some of the warm-up moves as fast as you can. Time yourself and try to beat your time each round. You can do it!

MENU

Breakfast:

Mexican Scrambled Eggs with Jalapeños, Tomatoes & Coriander *(see p88)*

Lunch:

Cottage Pie with Root Veg Mash *(defrosted from Day 9)*

Dinner:

Pork & Peanut Casserole *(see p146)*

Plus:

Chocolate Bombs *(stored from Day 10)*

WORKOUT

⭐ SATURDAY CHALLENGE ⭐

💗 **Warm-Up** *(see pp190–3)*

As fast as you can:

– 20 Butt Kickers *(see p192)*
– 20 Squat & Reach Out *(see p193)*

🔄 **Repeat the challenge two more times**

🔽 **Stretches & Cool-Down** *(see pp214–7)*

GLASSES OF WATER ⬜ ⬜ ⬜ ⬜ ⬜ ⬜ ⬜ ⬜

HOURS OF SLEEP

PM					AM												PM			
7	8	9	10	11	12	1	2	3	4	5	6	7	8	9	10	11	12	1	2	3	4

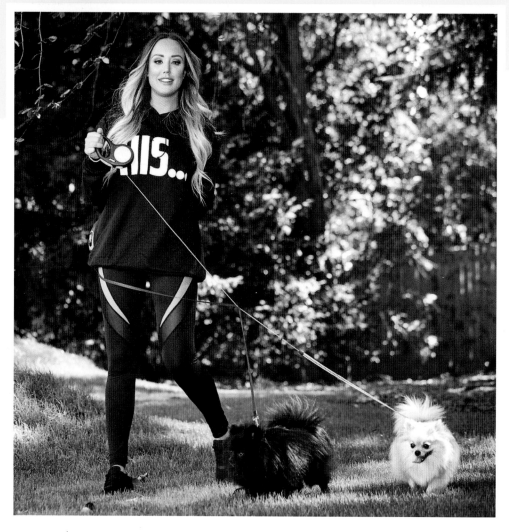

M T W T F S S

Today's fun time is about walking the dog. If you have your own dog (or three like me!) then think of it as your mini personal trainer because a dog is going to help you keep fit! If you haven't got a dog then don't let this minor fact deter you from going outside and looking the part – you can bring a toy one with you instead. Just tie a bit of string round its neck and whistle a lot. Don't forget to bring a carrier bag squashed up in one hand as if it's a poo bag. No one will ever know the difference…

MENU

Breakfast:

Full English Frittata *(see p86)*

Lunch:

Sweet Potato, Lentil & Spinach Soup
(see p127)

Dinner:

Roast Thai Salmon with Stir-Fried Veg & Rice Noodles
(see p142)

Plus:

Poached Pears with Vanilla Yoghurt *(see p172)*

WORKOUT

GO FOR A WALK*

*dogs optional

GLASSES OF WATER

HOURS OF SLEEP

PM   AM   PM

[7 | 8 | 9 | 10 | 11 | 12 | 1 | 2 | 3 | 4 | 5 | 6 | 7 | 8 | 9 | 10 | 11 | 12 | 1 | 2 | 3 | 4]

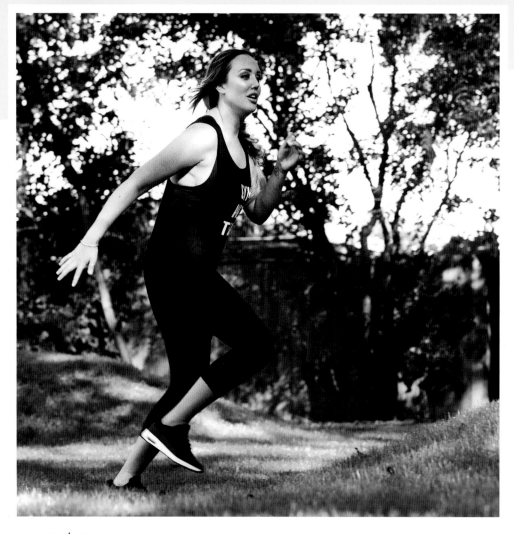

M T W T F S S

You've passed the halfway mark. This is quite an immense achievement! How have you done? How are you feeling? Is Monday feeling like a Saturday from all those exercise endorphins? Good! There are no Mondays in this new world! Every day is a Saturday remember! Saturdays are days of fun and laughter so there's no excuse not to have a big fat smile on your face. Even if it's raining run into your garden and get on with your workout!

MENU

Breakfast:

Home-made Baked Beans & Poached Eggs *(see p94)*

Lunch:

Roast Thai Salmon with Stir-Fried Veg & Rice Noodles *(leftover from Day 14)*

Dinner:

Lentil Ragu with Fresh Tomato Sauce & Courgetti Noodles *(see p138)*

Plus:

Protein Balls *(see p185)*

WORKOUT

🫀 **Warm-Up** *(see pp190–3)*

Do 35 seconds each of the following:

– Spidy Step & Reach *(see pp194–5)*
– Skywalkers *(see pp196–7)*
– Cowgirl Burpees *(see pp198–9)*
– Box Knee & Kick Out *(see pp200–1)*
– Star Jump & Front Kick *(see pp202–3)*
– Crunch & Alt Knee *(see pp204–5)*
– Lateral Jabs & Jacks *(see pp208–9)*
– Super Core Reach *(see pp210–11)*

🔄 **Repeat the workout two more times**

🧘 **Stretches & Cool-Down** *(see pp214–7)*

GLASSES of WATER

HOURS of SLEEP

| PM | | | | | AM | | | | | | | | | | | | PM | | | | |
| 7 | 8 | 9 | 10 | 11 | 12 | 1 | 2 | 3 | 4 | 5 | 6 | 7 | 8 | 9 | 10 | 11 | 12 | 1 | 2 | 3 | 4 |

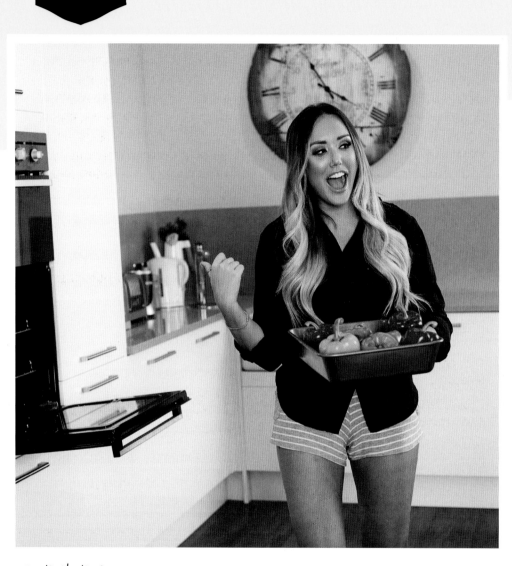

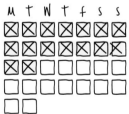

Sometimes I just like to fling something in the oven! By that I mean food, not a shoe or me mam. And while you're flinging things it's time to look at your clothes and be honest with yourself. 'Do I really need that top that looks like something me nana would wear?' Yes, it's time to blitz your wardrobe. If you haven't worn it in the last 18 months it needs to go! Also, this is a good excuse to chuck out those fat clothes you have – the ones you always wear when you hate your body – because you won't be needing them after the 30-Day Blitz!

MENU

Breakfast:

Mexican Omelette *(see p107)*

Lunch:

Lentil Ragu Stuffed Peppers *(see p112)*

Dinner:

Butternut Squash Pappardelle with Ricotta, Sage & Pine Nuts *(see p166)*

Plus:

Poached Pears with Vanilla Yoghurt *(see p172)*

WORKOUT

💜 **Warm-Up** *(see pp190–3)*

Do 35 seconds each of the following:

– Spidy Step & Reach *(see pp194–5)*
– Skywalkers *(see pp196–7)*
– Cowgirl Burpees *(see pp198–9)*
– Box Knee & Kick Out *(see pp200–1)*
– Star Jump & Front Kick *(see pp202–3)*
– Crunch & Alt Knee *(see pp204–5)*
– Lateral Jabs & Jacks *(see pp208–9)*
– Super Core Reach *(see pp210–11)*

🔄 **Repeat the workout two more times**

🧘 **Stretches & Cool-Down** *(see pp214–7)*

GLASSES OF WATER

HOURS OF SLEEP

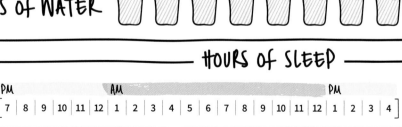

PM | AM | PM
[7 | 8 | 9 | 10 | 11 | 12 | 1 | 2 | 3 | 4 | 5 | 6 | 7 | 8 | 9 | 10 | 11 | 12 | 1 | 2 | 3 | 4]

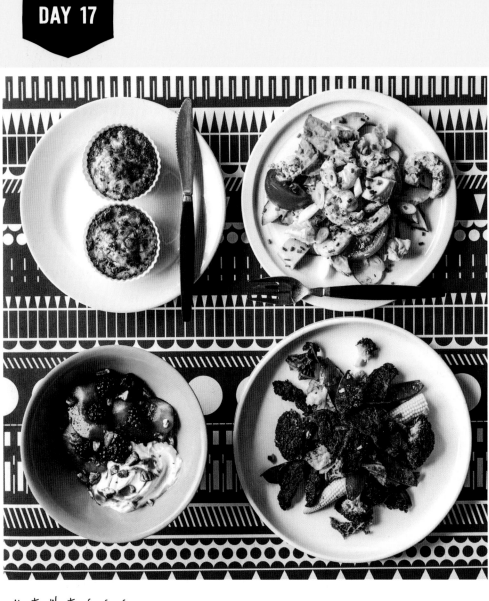

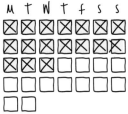

I've learnt that eating proper balanced meals with all the different food groups covered means your body never gets sick of anything and it feels much happier as a result! Doesn't this photo of everything you're going to eat today look amazing? It's like a Picasso painting (not that I've ever seen a Picasso painting but it sounds like it would be very pretty).

MENU

Breakfast:

All-in-One Baked Egg Cups
(see p96)

Lunch:

Prawn Cocktail Salad
(see p118)

Dinner:

Crispy Chilli Beef Stir Fry
with Loads of Veggies
(see p162)

Plus:

Baked Apple & Blackberry
with Maple Syrup Yoghurt
(see p174)

WORKOUT

♡ Warm-Up *(see pp190–3)*

Do 35 seconds each of the following:

– Spidy Step & Reach *(see pp194–5)*
– Skywalkers *(see pp196–7)*
– Cowgirl Burpees *(see pp198–9)*
– Box Knee & Kick Out *(see pp200–1)*
– Star Jump & Front Kick *(see pp202–3)*
– Crunch & Alt Knee *(see pp204–5)*
– Lateral Jabs & Jacks *(see pp208–9)*
– Super Core Reach *(see pp210–11)*

⚙ Repeat the workout two more times

⚕ Stretches & Cool-Down *(see pp214–7)*

GLASSES OF WATER

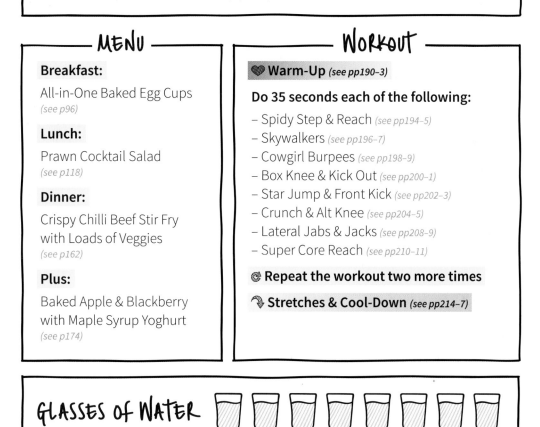

HOURS OF SLEEP

| PM | | | | | AM | | | | | | | | | | PM | | | | |
| 7 | 8 | 9 | 10 | 11 | 12 | 1 | 2 | 3 | 4 | 5 | 6 | 7 | 8 | 9 | 10 | 11 | 12 | 1 | 2 | 3 | 4 |

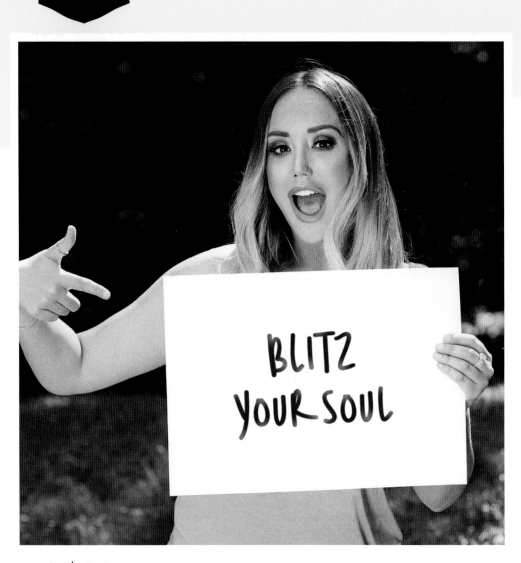

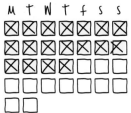

Blitz your soul. Maybe say a prayer or meditate. If there's something bad about your personality, today's the day to begin trying to get rid of it. (Obviously something as big and fundamental as a glitch in your character isn't going to be resolved in one day – but you can make a start!) I can be a bit short-tempered sometimes and always think I'm right. I don't let anyone else have a say. I am too quick to get angry and don't listen to the other person. So I am trying to get a grip on all of these things…

MENU

Breakfast:
Boiled Eggs with Rye Crispbread Toasts *(see p100)*

Lunch:
Red Lentil, Pepper & Chorizo Soup *(defrosted from Day 12)*

Dinner:
Wholewheat Pasta with Mixed Veg Sauce *(see p147)*

Plus:
Protein Balls *(stored from Day 15)*

WORKOUT

♥ **Warm-Up** *(see pp190–3)*

Do 35 seconds each of the following:
– Spidy Step & Reach *(see pp194–5)*
– Skywalkers *(see pp196–7)*
– Cowgirl Burpees *(see pp198–9)*
– Box Knee & Kick Out *(see pp200–1)*
– Star Jump & Front Kick *(see pp202–3)*
– Crunch & Alt Knee *(see pp204–5)*
– Lateral Jabs & Jacks *(see pp208–9)*
– Super Core Reach *(see pp210–11)*

⟳ **Repeat the workout two more times**

⟲ **Stretches & Cool-Down** *(see pp214–7)*

GLASSES of WATER

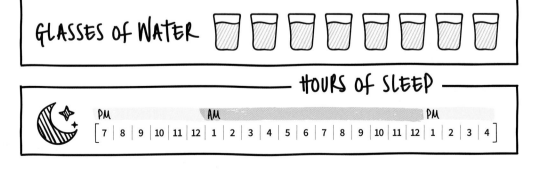

HOURS of SLEEP

PM — AM — PM
[7 | 8 | 9 | 10 | 11 | 12 | 1 | 2 | 3 | 4 | 5 | 6 | 7 | 8 | 9 | 10 | 11 | 12 | 1 | 2 | 3 | 4]

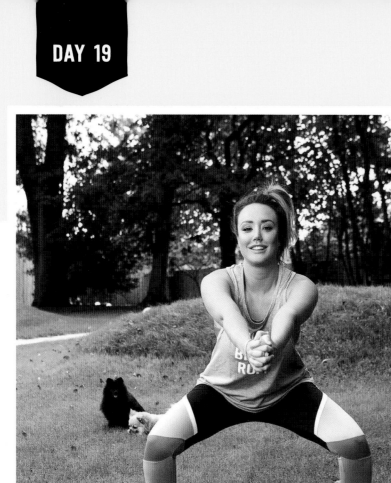

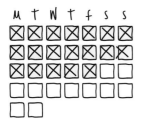

Exercise doesn't have to happen at a strict time of day – everyone is different and has different times that work better for them. You might find it easier in the morning (and it's out of the way then) or you might be an evening type person (so do some sit-ups in front of the telly). Or, you might be the sort of person who looks like they are pooing a couple of dogs out of their bum like I do in this picture of me doing a squat in the garden! Whatever suits you, as long as you do it!

MENU

Breakfast:

Green Smoothie
with Greek Yoghurt *(see p90)*

Lunch:

Wholewheat Pasta
with Mixed Veg Sauce
(leftover from Day 18)

Dinner:

Chicken Nuggets &
Sweet Potato Chips *(see p137)*

Plus:

Smoked Trout Pâté
with Veg Sticks *(see p184)*

WORKOUT

♥ **Warm-Up** *(see pp190–3)*

Do 35 seconds each of the following:

– Spidy Step & Reach *(see pp194–5)*
– Skywalkers *(see pp196–7)*
– Cowgirl Burpees *(see pp198–9)*
– Box Knee & Kick Out *(see pp200–1)*
– Star Jump & Front Kick *(see pp202–3)*
– Crunch & Alt Knee *(see pp204–5)*
– Lateral Jabs & Jacks *(see pp208–9)*
– Super Core Reach *(see pp210–11)*

🌀 **Repeat the workout two more times**

🐍 **Stretches & Cool-Down** *(see pp214–7)*

GLASSES OF WATER

HOURS OF SLEEP

PM					AM											PM			
7	8	9	10	11	12	1	2	3	4	5	6	7	8	9	10	11	12	1	2	3	4

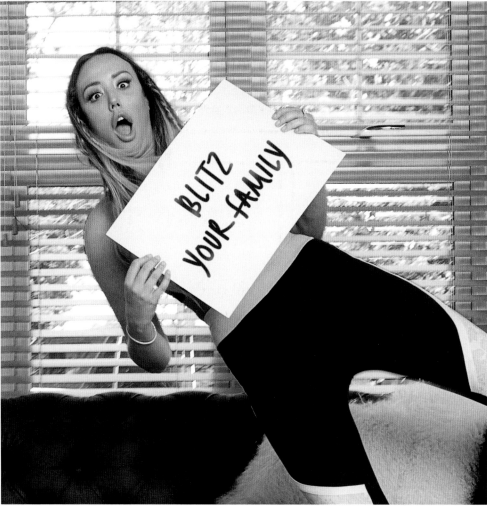

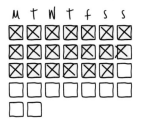

Blitz your family. By that I mean blitz them with love! It's Saturday so take them somewhere bonding and nice like the cinema or bowling. Me and my family always go bowling. I always get very competitive. Nathaniel should be rubbish because he's the youngest but he gets to have the crash barriers up so he always does OK. You could get them to try the challenge too, you could even set up a scoreboard, if you're feeling especially competitve.

MENU

Breakfast:
Baked Egg Pots *(see p101)*

Lunch:
Red Lentil, Pepper
& Chorizo Soup
(see p126)

Dinner:
Roast Turmeric Cauliflower
& Lamb Curry with Wild Rice
(see p140)

Plus:
Berry Frozen Yoghurt
(stored in the freezer from Day 4)

WORKOUT

⭐ SATURDAY CHALLENGE ⭐

💙 **Warm-Up** *(see pp190–3)*

As fast as you can:
– 20 Mountain Climbers *(see p206–7)*
– 20 Butt Kickers *(see p192)*
– 20 Squat & Reach Out *(see p193)*

🔄 **Repeat the challenge two more times**

🌿 **Stretches & Cool-Down** *(see pp214–7)*

GLASSES of WATER

HOURS of SLEEP

PM | AM | PM
[7 | 8 | 9 | 10 | 11 | 12 | 1 | 2 | 3 | 4 | 5 | 6 | 7 | 8 | 9 | 10 | 11 | 12 | 1 | 2 | 3 | 4]

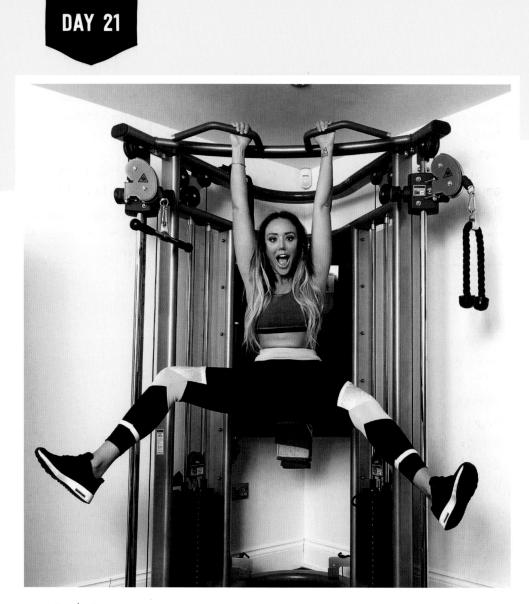

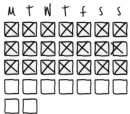

It's fun time Sunday! Ring or call in to your local gym and find out if you can have a free trial or a guest pass for the day (they like to give them away to tempt you to join) or ask a friend who is already a member if they have any free passes. Book a nice treatment for yourself in their spa or get your make-up or nails done and make a day of it with one of your mates. If your friends are anything like mine then you will end up laughing all day, which will have the added bonus of working your stomach muscles!

MENU

Breakfast:
Breakfast Tray Bake *(see p95)*

Lunch:
All Green Soup
(see p114)

Dinner:
Roasted Salmon with Slaw
in Citrus Dressing *(see p136)*

Plus:
Poached Pears
with Vanilla Yoghurt *(see p172)*

WORKOUT

TRY OUT A GYM

GLASSES OF WATER

HOURS OF SLEEP

	PM					AM											PM			
7	8	9	10	11	12	1	2	3	4	5	6	7	8	9	10	11	12	1	2	3	4

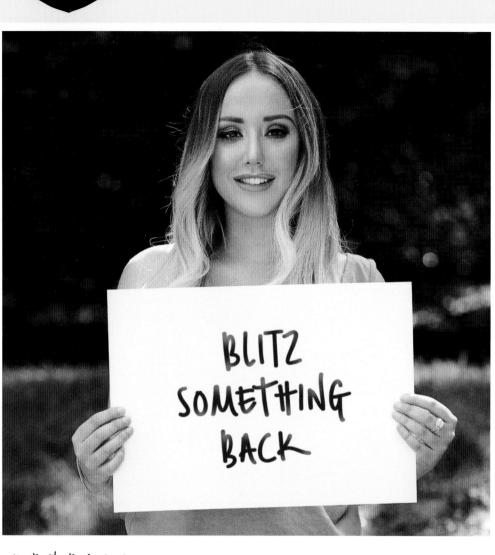

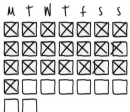

Blitz something back. Try to make a positive difference to other people's lives; always give back to the world in any way you can. There are a lot of different charities I support that are close to my heart – like the National Autistic Society; Barnardos; The Make a Wish Foundation; Animal Welfare Queensland and the St John and Elizabeth Hospice. I am a Patron of the Ectopic Pregnancy Trust following my awful experience in 2016. Think about the charity you'd like help and ways you can fund-raise or support it.

MENU

Breakfast:

Herby Falafel Waffles with Poached Eggs *(defrost waffles from Day 3, see pp92–3 for the eggs)*

Lunch:

Roasted Salmon with Slaw in Citrus Dressing

(leftover from Day 21)

Dinner:

Shredded Chicken Noodle Soup with Sweet Potato Noodles *(see p141)*

Plus:

Spiced Nuts *(see p186)*

WORKOUT

💙 **Warm-Up** *(see pp190–3)*

Do 40 seconds each of the following:

– Super Core Reach *(see pp210–11)*
– Lateral Jabs & Jacks *(see pp208–9)*
– Crunch & Alt Knee *(see pp204–5)*
– Star Jump & Front Kick *(see pp202–3)*
– Box Knee & Kick Out *(see pp200–1)*
– Cowgirl Burpees *(see pp198–9)*
– Skywalkers *(see pp196–7)*
– Spidy Step & Reach *(see pp194–5)*
– Alternate Lunges & Wood Chops *(see pp212–3)*

🌀 **Repeat the workout two more times**

🏃 **Stretches & Cool-Down** *(see pp214–7)*

GLASSES OF WATER

HOURS OF SLEEP

PM					AM											PM					
7	8	9	10	11	12	1	2	3	4	5	6	7	8	9	10	11	12	1	2	3	4

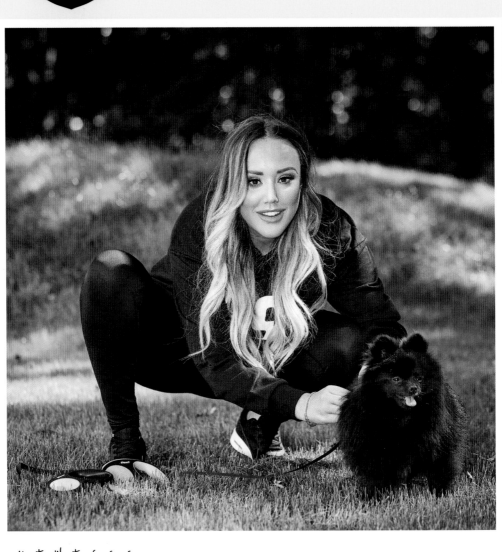

M T W T F S S
☒ ☒ ☒ ☒ ☒ ☒ ☒
☒ ☒ ☒ ☒ ☒ ☒ ☒
☒ ☒ ☒ ☒ ☒ ☒ ☒
☒ ☒ ☐ ☐ ☐ ☐ ☐
☐ ☐

Blitz your pets (again don't read this wrong and think I mean get rid of them – like the family blitz, this blitz all comes from your love and affection for those furry things). If you've got a rabbit, clean the hutch. If you have goldfish, wash out the bowl. And if you have dogs, give them a bath. I am quite used to shoving Rhubarb in the bath and hosing her with the shower because she always ends up covered in poo, so even though it's rank I do my bit.

MENU

Breakfast:

Protein Packed Omelette
(see p107)

Lunch:

Shredded Chicken Noodle Soup with Sweet Potato Noodles
(leftover from Day 22)

Dinner:

Vegetable Lasagne
(see p152)

Plus:

Spiced Nuts *(stored from Day 22)*

WORKOUT

💗 **Warm-Up** *(see pp190–3)*

Do 40 seconds each of the following:

– Super Core Reach *(see pp210–11)*
– Lateral Jabs & Jacks *(see pp208–9)*
– Crunch & Alt Knee *(see pp204–5)*
– Star Jump & Front Kick *(see pp202–3)*
– Box Knee & Kick Out *(see pp200–1)*
– Cowgirl Burpees *(see pp198–9)*
– Skywalkers *(see pp196–7)*
– Spidy Step & Reach *(see pp194–5)*
– Alternate Lunges & Wood Chops *(see pp212–3)*

🔄 **Repeat the workout two more times**

🏃 **Stretches & Cool-Down** *(see pp214–7)*

GLASSES of WATER

HOURS of SLEEP

PM   AM   PM

[7 | 8 | 9 | 10 | 11 | 12 | 1 | 2 | 3 | 4 | 5 | 6 | 7 | 8 | 9 | 10 | 11 | 12 | 1 | 2 | 3 | 4]

DAY 24

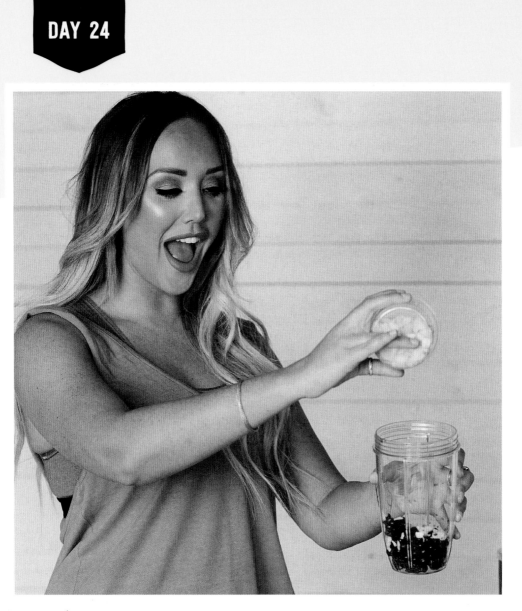

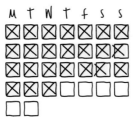

Blitz a smoothie. A recipe in the Blitz where you actually get to blitz! It's much better (and more fun) to make a smoothie at home because not all smoothies are goodies – watch out for the ones you get in supermarkets as they can look like they are healthy but often have loads of sugar hidden in them. So beware the danger drink!

MENU

Breakfast:

Almond and Berry Smoothie
(see p104)

Lunch:

Vegetable Lasagne
(leftover from Day 23)

Dinner:

Crispy Coconut Cod
with Pineapple Rice *(see p157)*

Plus:

Vegetable Crisps *(see p178)*

WORKOUT

💜 **Warm-Up** *(see pp190–3)*

Do 40 seconds each of the following:

– Super Core Reach *(see pp210–11)*
– Lateral Jabs & Jacks *(see pp208–9)*
– Crunch & Alt Knee *(see pp204–5)*
– Star Jump & Front Kick *(see pp202–3)*
– Box Knee & Kick Out *(see pp200–1)*
– Cowgirl Burpees *(see pp198–9)*
– Skywalkers *(see pp196–7)*
– Spidy Step & Reach *(see pp194–5)*
– Alternate Lunges & Wood Chops
  (see pp212–3)

🌀 **Repeat the workout two more times**

🍃 **Stretches & Cool-Down** *(see pp214–7)*

WATER

HOURS OF SLEEP

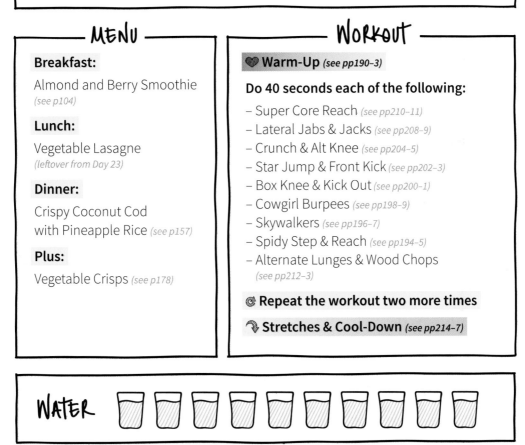

| PM | | | | | | AM | | | | | | | | | | | | PM | | | |
| 7 | 8 | 9 | 10 | 11 | 12 | 1 | 2 | 3 | 4 | 5 | 6 | 7 | 8 | 9 | 10 | 11 | 12 | 1 | 2 | 3 | 4 |

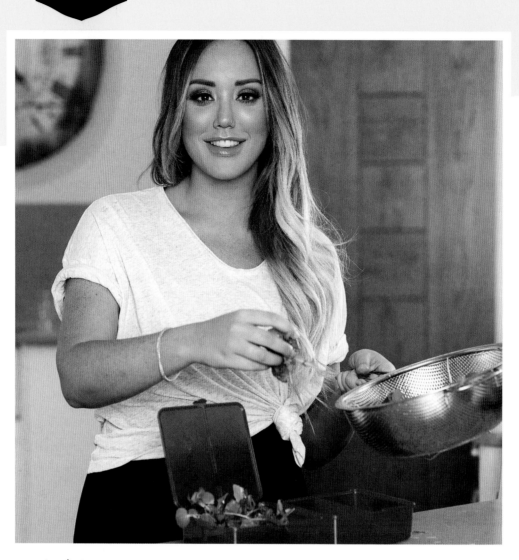

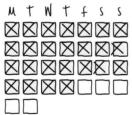

Taking your own lunch to work will become the best habit you ever formed. I always take a load of green salad leaves – what could be quicker than throwing some green things in a box?! For starters you will save loads of money because you won't be tempted to buy the whole sandwich shelf in M&S. And even better, it's really easy and healthy. Fill a box to go with these fritters.

MENU

Breakfast:

Boiled Eggs with Rye Crispbread Toasts *(see p100)*

Lunch:

Chickpea & Jalapeño Fritters with Feta Dip & Roast Tomatoes *(see p120)*

Dinner:

Crispy Chilli Beef Stir Fry with Loads of Veggies *(see p162)*

Plus:

Vegetable Crisps *(stored from Day 24)*

WORKOUT

♥ Warm-Up *(see pp190–3)*

Do 40 seconds each of the following:

– Super Core Reach *(see pp210–11)*
– Lateral Jabs & Jacks *(see pp208–9)*
– Crunch & Alt Knee *(see pp204–5)*
– Star Jump & Front Kick *(see pp202–3)*
– Box Knee & Kick Out *(see pp200–1)*
– Cowgirl Burpees *(see pp198–9)*
– Skywalkers *(see pp196–7)*
– Spidy Step & Reach *(see pp194–5)*
– Alternate Lunges & Wood Chops *(see pp212–3)*

↻ Repeat the workout two more times

↝ Stretches & Cool-Down *(see pp214–7)*

GLASSES of WATER

HOURS of SLEEP

PM — AM — PM
[7 | 8 | 9 | 10 | 11 | 12 | 1 | 2 | 3 | 4 | 5 | 6 | 7 | 8 | 9 | 10 | 11 | 12 | 1 | 2 | 3 | 4]

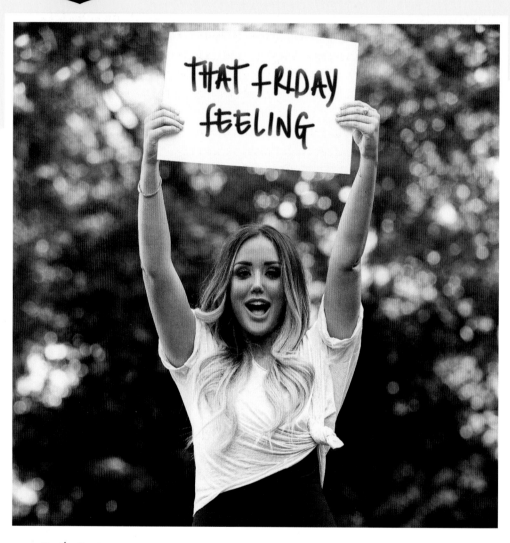

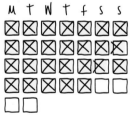

It's Friday which means you're at the end of another successful week – take a good Friday look at yourself in the mirror and flick your hair in a Friday way! Today it's time to blitz your car. Throw out those crisp packets, old brown apple cores under the seat, half-read magazines, the odd hair extension and that earring you have been looking for since last Christmas… chuck them! And get the portable Hoover out this minute! Don't have a car? Blitz someone else's!

MENU

Breakfast:

Herby Falafel Waffles with Poached Eggs *(defrost waffles from Day 3, see pp92–3 for the eggs)*

Lunch:

Grilled Salmon with Italian Courgette Salad *(see p115)*

Dinner:

Turkey Chilli con Carne with Shredded Green Veg *(defrosted from Day 5)*

Plus:

Vegetable Crisps *(stored from Day 24)*

WORKOUT

💗 **Warm-Up** *(see pp190–3)*

Do 40 seconds each of the following:

– Super Core Reach *(see pp210–11)*
– Lateral Jabs & Jacks *(see pp208–9)*
– Crunch & Alt Knee *(see pp204–5)*
– Star Jump & Front Kick *(see pp202–3)*
– Box Knee & Kick Out *(see pp200–1)*
– Cowgirl Burpees *(see pp198–9)*
– Skywalkers *(see pp196–7)*
– Spidy Step & Reach *(see pp194–5)*
– Alternate Lunges & Wood Chops *(see pp212–3)*

🌀 **Repeat the workout two more times**

🐾 **Stretches & Cool-Down** *(see pp214–7)*

GLASSES of WATER

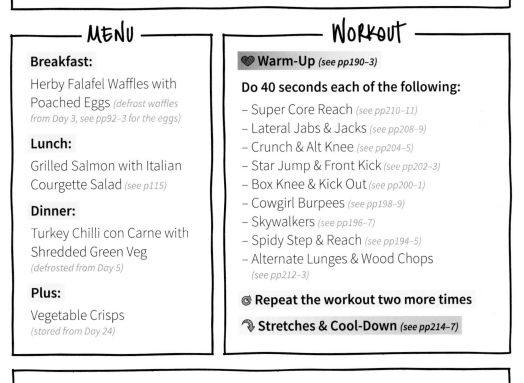

HOURS of SLEEP

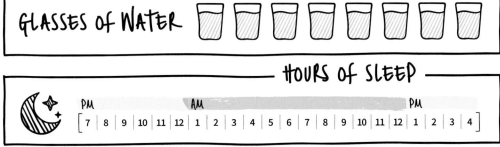

| PM | | | | | AM | | | | | | | | | | | PM | | | |
| 7 | 8 | 9 | 10 | 11 | 12 | 1 | 2 | 3 | 4 | 5 | 6 | 7 | 8 | 9 | 10 | 11 | 12 | 1 | 2 | 3 | 4 |

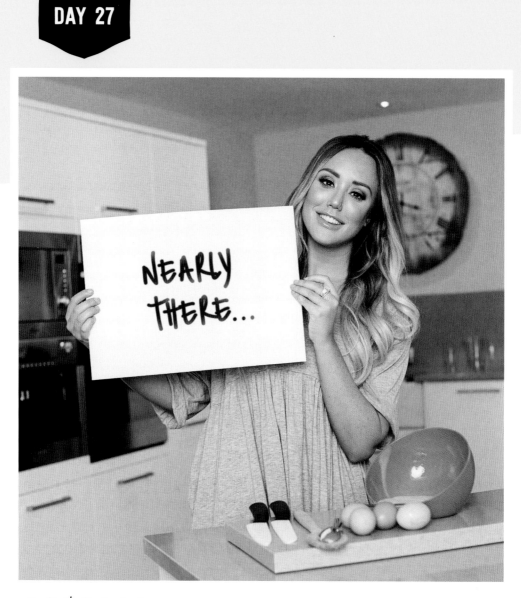

M T W T F S S

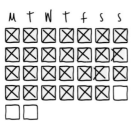

This is your last Saturday of the challenge so it's definitely one you should get friends round for. Invite your mates over and make them paella (they will be VERY impressed with your skills). They will be even more impressed that these Chocolate Bombs are actually part of the Blitz. Just because you're on a blitz doesn't mean you can't have fun. Or any friends!

MENU

Breakfast:
Vegetable Omelette *(see p106)*

Lunch:
Rainbow Noodles with Sweet & Spicy Sauce *(see p110)*

Dinner:
Seafood Paella *(see p148)*

Plus:
Chocolate Bombs *(see p173)*

WORKOUT

⭐ SATURDAY CHALLENGE ⭐

💗 **Warm-Up** *(see pp190–3)*

As fast as you can:
– 20 Mountain Climbers *(see pp206–7)*
– 20 Butt Kickers *(see p192)*
– 20 Squat & Reach Out *(see p193)*
– 20 Lateral Jabs & Jacks *(see pp208–9)*

🔄 **Repeat the challenge**

🌀 **Stretches & Cool-Down** *(see pp214–7)*

GLASSES of WATER

HOURS of SLEEP

PM					AM												PM			
7	8	9	10	11	12	1	2	3	4	5	6	7	8	9	10	11	12	1	2	3	4

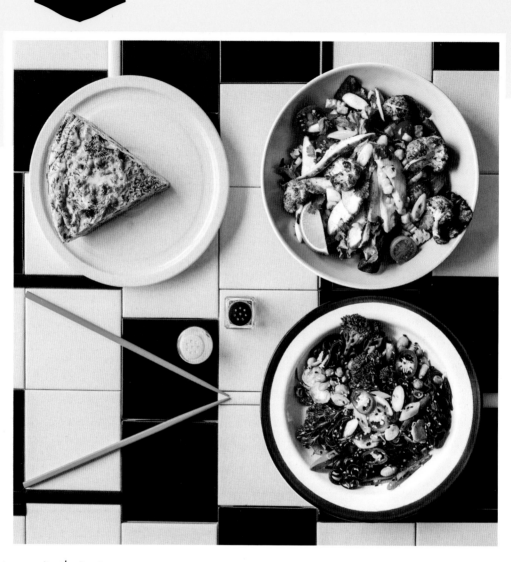

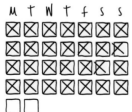

Let's make the last Sunday amazing. Do something you know you wouldn't have been able to do before – run up and down the stairs, run faster and longer than you usually do. You're feeling so much better in mind and body… make it count in every part of your life! And for the final blitz… blitz your partner. It's time to get any issues off your chest. Even if they are just small problems then it's best to talk about them and if you are happy about everything in your relationship tell them that too. And maybe treat them to some H.I.F..

MENU

Breakfast:

Full English Frittata *(see p86)*

Lunch:

Grillled Corn, Avocado & Chilli Chicken Salad *(see p128)*

Dinner:

Black Rice Noodles with Greens & Sesame Seeds *(see p154)*

Plus:

Poached Pears with Vanilla Yoghurt *(see p172)*

WORKOUT

GO FOR A RUN

GLASSES OF WATER

HOURS OF SLEEP

PM   AM   PM

[7 | 8 | 9 | 10 | 11 | 12 | 1 | 2 | 3 | 4 | 5 | 6 | 7 | 8 | 9 | 10 | 11 | 12 | 1 | 2 | 3 | 4]

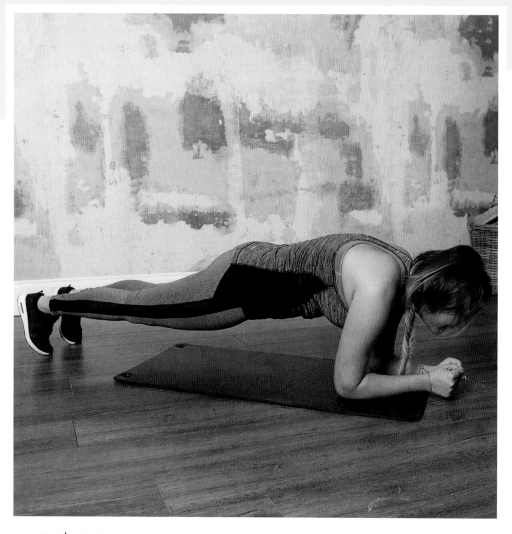

M T W T F S S
⊠⊠⊠⊠⊠⊠⊠
⊠⊠⊠⊠⊠⊠⊠
⊠⊠⊠⊠⊠⊠⊠
⊠⊠⊠⊠⊠⊠⊠
⊠☐

Only one more day to go. I can hardly believe it! What are we going to do with ourselves? I'm going to miss bossing you about. I might have to start it all over again next month! But before you go it's time for the final challenge. Try to hold the plank for at least 20 seconds. Just don't forget to breathe. I don't want you to die when we've got this far. That would make me very upset (and wouldn't be good for my reputation).

MENU

Breakfast:

Coconut Pancakes with Mango & Lime Yoghurt
(defrosted from Day 6)

Lunch:

Red Lentil, Pepper & Chorizo Soup
(defrosted from Day 20)

Dinner:

Pork & Peanut Casserole
(defrosted from Day 13)

Plus:

Baked Apple & Blackberry with Maple Syrup Yoghurt
(see p174)

WORKOUT

FINAL CHALLENGE

🧡 **Warm-Up** *(see pp190–3)*

Hold a plank *(see p197)* **for 20 seconds**

As fast as you can:

– 20 Mountain Climbers *(see pp206–7)*
– 20 Butt Kickers *(see p192)*
– 20 Squat & Reach Out *(see p193)*
– 20 Lateral Jabs & Jacks *(see pp208–9)*

〰️ **Stretches & Cool-Down** *(see pp214–7)*

GLASSES of WATER

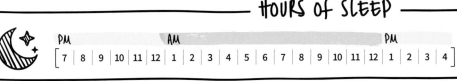

HOURS of SLEEP

PM					AM												PM			
7	8	9	10	11	12	1	2	3	4	5	6	7	8	9	10	11	12	1	2	3	4

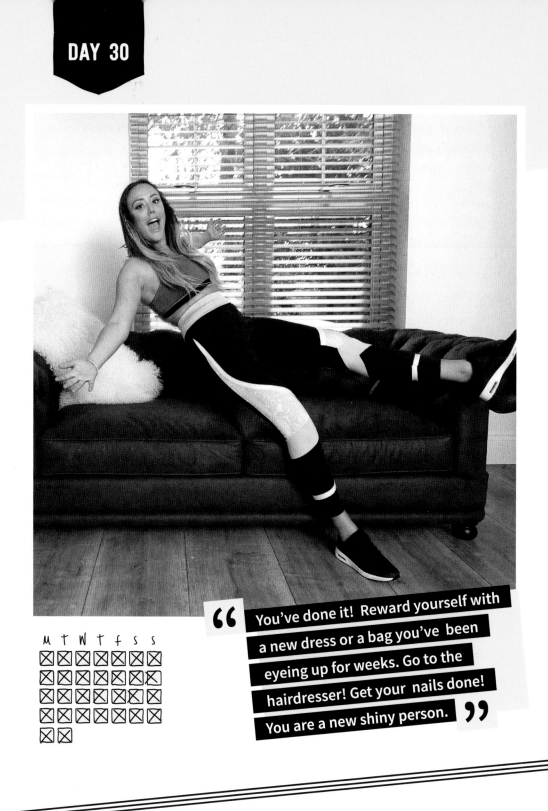

M T W T F S S

☒ ☒ ☒ ☒ ☒ ☒ ☒
☒ ☒ ☒ ☒ ☒ ☒ ☒
☒ ☒ ☒ ☒ ☒ ☒ ☒
☒ ☒ ☒ ☒ ☒ ☒ ☒
☒ ☒

" You've done it! Reward yourself with a new dress or a bag you've been eyeing up for weeks. Go to the hairdresser! Get your nails done! You are a new shiny person. "

Massive well done and a big high-five for reaching Day 30. It's time to reward yourself. You are a shiny new person, so don't wipe that smile off your face all day. Think about what you've achieved and how much fitter, stronger and leaner you are. Don't go back to bad ways! You've still got food in the fridge and freezer, and you can do these workouts any time – keep it up and you will continue to feel amazing. Let me know how you are getting on!

MENU

Breakfast:

Home-made Baked Beans & Poached Eggs *(see p94)*

Lunch:

Vegetable Lasagne
(defrosted from Day 23)

Dinner:

Sweet Potato Noodle Pad Thai *(see p132)*

Plus:

Spiced Nuts *(stored from Day 22)*

GLASSES OF WATER

WORKOUT

🫀 **Warm-Up** *(see pp190–3)*

Do 20 seconds each of the following, with a lunge and chop between each exercise (alternating left and right legs with each exercise):

– Spidy Step & Reach *(see pp194–5)*
– Skywalkers *(see pp196–7)*
– Cowgirl Burpees *(see pp198–9)*
– Box Knee & Kick Out *(see pp200–1)*
– Star Jump & Front Kick *(see pp202–3)*
– Crunch & Alt Knee *(see pp204–5)*
– Lateral Jabs & Jacks *(see pp208–9)*
– Super Core Reach *(see pp210–11)*

Rest for 1 minute, then repeat in reverse order doing each exercise for 25 seconds followed by the lunge and chop.

♺ **Repeat the whole workout but with no rest**

🍃 **Stretches & Cool-Down** *(see pp214–7)*

FINAL WORKOUT

HOURS OF SLEEP

PM					AM											PM			
7	8	9	10	11	12	1	2	3	4	5	6	7	8	9	10	11	12	1	2	3	4

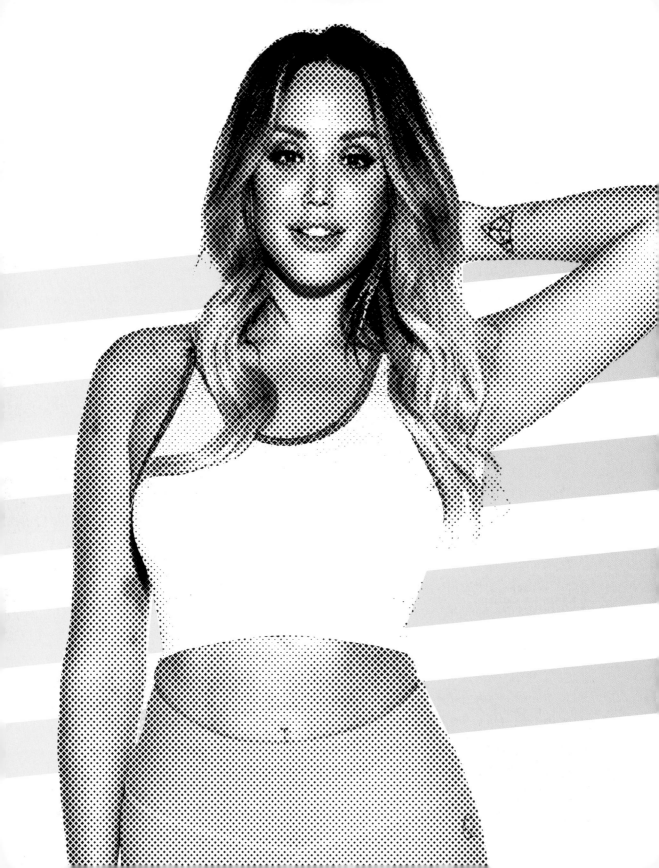

RECIPES

BREAK -FAST

I won't be the first person to tell you that this is the most important meal of the day. Make breakfast your boyfriend and tell it how much you love it every morning.

FULL ENGLISH FRITTATA
Serves 4–6

I think 'frittata' is a brilliant word (nearly as good as guacamole). It would make quite a good name for a girl: 'Hi, my name's Frittata Crosby – how are you? Don't try and eat me please.'

1 tbsp rapeseed oil

1 onion, peeled and roughly chopped

4 rashers back bacon, excess fat trimmed, cut into pieces (about 25g each once fat has been removed)

2 pork sausages, at least 97% pork, each cut into 8 pieces (about 55g each)

2 tomatoes, each cut into 6 wedges (about 85g each)

6 chestnut mushrooms, sliced

8 medium free-range eggs

10g fresh chives, roughly chopped

4 portions of Home-made Baked Beans (see page 94)

- Preheat the oven to 170°C/150°C fan/gas 3.
- Heat the oil in an ovenproof non-stick frying pan over a medium heat. If you don't have an ovenproof frying pan, use a regular frying pan and then transfer the mixture to a lined cake tin or small roasting tin before adding the eggs instead.
- Fry the onion, bacon and sausage together in the pan for about 8–10 minutes, or until the onion starts to go golden brown. Add the tomatoes and mushrooms and continue to cook for another 5 minutes.
- Crack the eggs into a jug and beat them with a fork or whisk. Add the chives and pour 80% of the mixture into the frying pan, turning off the heat. Stir everything well to make sure the eggs go all around the other ingredients. Spoon the home-made baked beans into the frittata in dollops.
- Finally, pour the last of the egg mixture over the top of everything in the pan to seal it. Put the whole pan into the oven and bake for 20–25 minutes, or until the frittata has risen slightly and is golden brown.
- Remove from the oven and leave to cool in the pan for 10 minutes, then slide out onto a chopping board. Slice, serve and eat straight away, or allow to cool and take with you for breakfast on the go.

MAKE IT VEGGIE: Swap the pork sausages for a vegetarian alternative (but check the labels because they can be salty), scrap the bacon and add another six mushrooms and a couple of handfuls of spinach (frozen is fine).

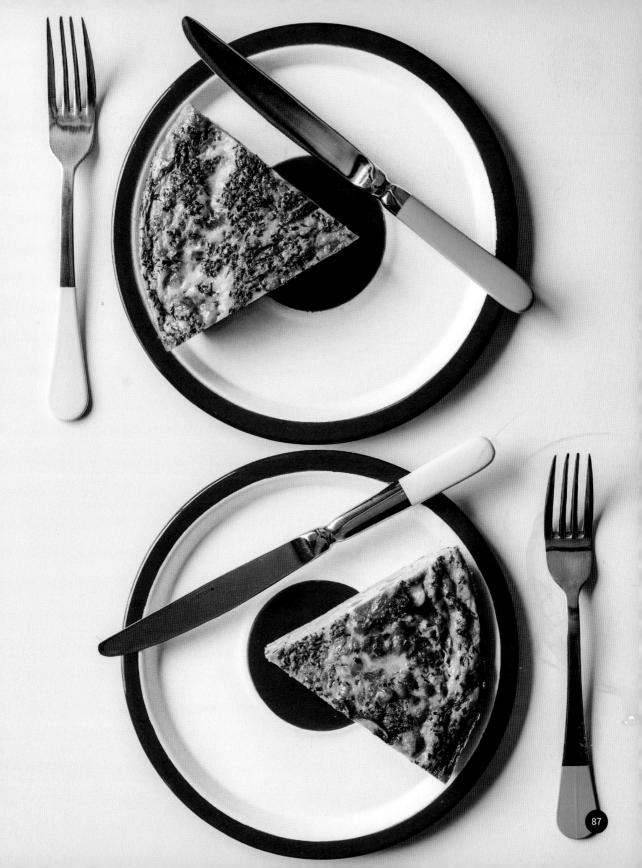

MEXICAN SCRAMBLED EGGS WITH JALAPEÑOS, TOMATOES & CORIANDER

Serves 2

Check out this baby – it's not only filling but its soooo tasty. I told you breakfasts were the best. And if you haven't been converted to Tabasco yet you will soon become an addict. Hot hot hot!

4 medium free-range eggs
5g unsalted butter
1 banana shallot, peeled and finely chopped
1 jalapeño, finely chopped (seeds removed if you prefer less heat)
12 cherry tomatoes, quartered
10g fresh coriander, roughly chopped
a few drops of Tabasco (optional)
salt and black pepper

- Crack the eggs into a mixing bowl and season to taste. Beat well with a fork and set aside.
- Heat the butter in a medium non-stick frying pan over a low heat. Once it's melted, add the shallot and jalapeño and cook for about 3–4 minutes, stirring often to cook evenly.
- Add the tomatoes and cook for another 2 minutes, until they just start to break down.
- Add the eggs and stir to mix everything together. Keep the eggs moving gently over the heat.
- Add the chopped coriander, keeping some to one side for garnish, and continue cooking.
- Once the eggs are cooked to your liking, divide them between two plates. Add a few drops of Tabasco, if you're using it, and some coriander leaves to garnish.

TIP: A low heat and slow cooking make delicious creamy scrambled eggs, so try not to rush this.

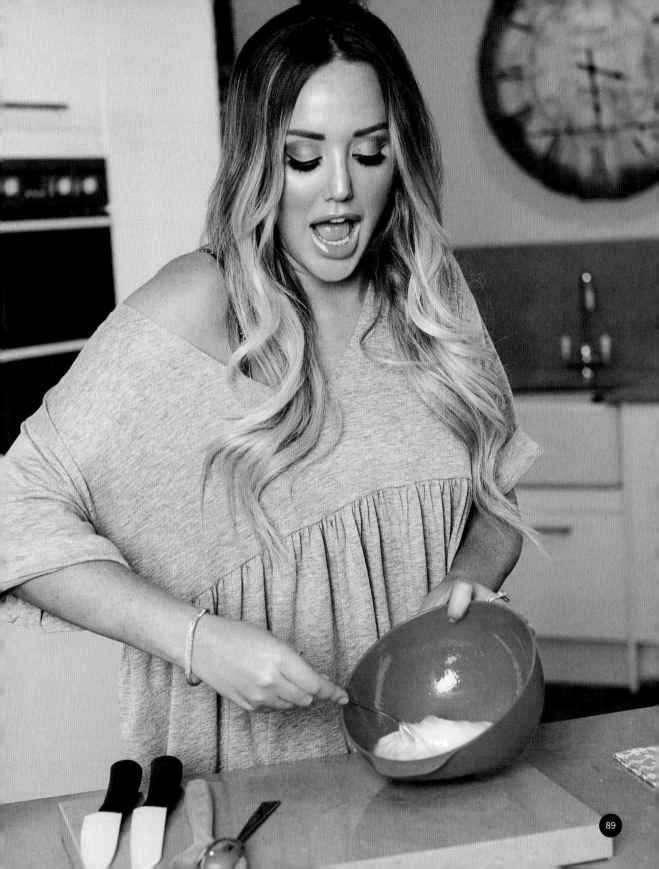

GREEN SMOOTHIE WITH GREEK YOGHURT

Serves 2

This is a smoothie with mean power. That's because it's green. and everyone knows that green things are good for you.

300ml 0% fat natural
Greek-style yoghurt
100g spinach or baby
spinach, washed and
roughly chopped
200g cucumber,
roughly chopped
1 Granny Smith apple, cored
40g almonds, blanched
1 lime, juice only (more if
you like it zingier)
a few fresh mint leaves

• Tip all the ingredients, apart from the mint, into a blender with 200ml of water and blitz for 4–5 minutes until it is really smooth. If it's too thick for you, just add a splash more water.
• Serve in large glasses with ice and some fresh mint leaves.

OVERNIGHT PEANUT BUTTER OATS WITH APPLE SLICES

Serves 2

I cannot tell you how amazingly yummy this tastes – it's worth the extra bit of effort to get it prepped overnight. You will never look back!

360ml semi-skimmed milk
4 tsp smooth peanut butter (choose one with no added anything)
100g gluten-free oats
2 tsp hemp protein powder
1 tsp ground cinnamon
2 Granny Smith apples
2 tbsp sultanas

- Divide the milk and peanut butter between two small-ish airtight containers or jars. Give them a little mix to mingle the ingredients.
- Leaving the peel on, core and grate the apple. Divide the oats, protein powder, cinnamon, apple and sultanas between the two jars and mix well. Make sure the oats are well covered in the milk before putting the lids on and popping them into the fridge overnight.
- In the morning slice up the other apple and divide between the two jars and enjoy. Easy peasy.

HERBY FALAFEL WAFFLES WITH POACHED EGGS

Serves 2

Waffles are wonderful. Waffles are wicked. Waffles are welcoming. Waffles are wobbly (if you try and wave one in the air). And these waffles are well healthy! (Do I need to point out that you need a waffle iron for this one?)

For the waffles

400g tin chickpeas, drained
2 banana shallots, peeled and roughly chopped
3 cloves garlic, peeled and roughly chopped
100g spinach or baby spinach, washed
20g fresh coriander
10g flat-leaf parsley
2 tsp ground cumin
1 tsp cayenne pepper
100g gluten-free self-raising flour
1 large free-range egg
80ml semi-skimmed milk
200g cherry tomatoes
¼ tsp coconut oil, for greasing
salt and black pepper

For the eggs

3 tbsp white wine vinegar
2 large free-range eggs

- Preheat the oven to 200°C/180°C fan/gas 6 and line a roasting tin with non-stick baking parchment.
- Place the chickpeas, shallots, garlic, spinach, fresh herbs, spices and flour into a food processor and blitz it all together into a paste. This will take a couple of minutes. Add the egg and milk and blitz again to form a thick batter. Season with salt and pepper if you wish and set aside.
- Put the cherry tomatoes into the roasting tin and cook in the oven for 15–20 minutes.
- Meanwhile, preheat the waffle iron to a medium-high setting. Use a pastry brush or kitchen paper and a little coconut oil to grease the waffle iron to prevent sticking.
- Add large spoonfuls of the batter to the waffle iron and use the back of the spoon to spread it out to fill the base. Cook for 8–10 minutes (you don't want the outside to burn before the inside is cooked through). Once it is golden brown, set aside and keep warm while you continue to cook the remaining batter.
- Meanwhile, bring a large saucepan of water to the boil. Add the vinegar to the pan and reduce the heat to a simmer. Using the end of a wooden spoon, stir to make a swirl in the water. While the water is

still spinning, crack the first egg in down the side of the pan (the water will pull the egg into the middle). Then crack in the second egg. Poach the eggs for 3 minutes for runny yolks, or up to 7 minutes for a well-done, firm yolk. Lift the eggs out with a slotted spoon and drain on kitchen paper.

- Serve one waffle per person, topped with an egg and with the roasted tomatoes on the side.
- Freeze the six remaining cooked waffles

TIP: When you freeze the waffles separate them with non-stick baking parchment before putting them in the freezer. Defrost overnight before you reheat them.

HOME-MADE BAKED BEANS & POACHED EGGS

Serves 2

If you're someone who loves baked beans then this is the recipe you need in your life. Tinned ones are full of sugar so this is the way to have them from now on. Just don't eat them all at once, make this recipe and you'll have leftovers for another day.

For the beans
1 tbsp olive oil
1 small onion, peeled
    and finely chopped
1 tbsp tomato purée
400g tin plum tomatoes
2 tbsp Worcestershire sauce
1 tbsp maple syrup
1 tbsp cider vinegar
1 tbsp smoked paprika
½ tbsp ground cumin
2 x 400g tins haricot beans,
    drained
salt and black pepper

For the eggs
3 tbsp white wine vinegar
2 large free-range eggs

To garnish
a handful of coriander
    leaves
4 spring onions, sliced

- To make the beans, heat the oil in a large saucepan over a medium heat and add the onion. Cook for 5 minutes, or until they start to soften and go golden. Add the tomato purée and stir through, then add the tomatoes. Add the Worcestershire sauce, maple syrup, cider vinegar and the spices. Let it all cook together for about 10 minutes, stirring occasionally. As it cooks, break the plum tomatoes open with the back of a wooden spoon.
- Once the sauce has thickened, which may take another 5–10 minutes, turn down the heat and add the haricot beans. Cook for 20 minutes over a low heat. Season with salt and pepper if you wish.
- Meanwhile, bring a large saucepan of water to the boil. Add the vinegar to the pan and reduce the heat to a simmer. Using the end of a wooden spoon, stir to make a swirl in the water. While the water is still spinning, crack in the first egg down the side of the pan (the water will pull the egg into the middle). Then crack in the second egg. Poach the eggs for 3 minutes for runny yolks, or up to 7 minutes for a well-done, firm yolk. Lift the eggs out with a slotted spoon and drain on kitchen paper.
- Spoon out two portions of beans and top each one with a poached egg. Garnish with the coriander leaves and spring onion and serve.

TIP: The beans will serve six so keep the leftovers in the fridge for up to four days in an airtight container. You can also use the leftovers in the Full English Frittata on page 86.

BREAKFAST TRAY BAKE

Serves 2

There is literally nothing not to like about this – it's a tray of dreams. It's so amazing all packed in together you will never miss toast. Toast is so last year – its all about trays!

1 **tsp** rapeseed oil
2 pork sausages, at least 97% pork (about 55g each)
2 tomatoes, halved (about 85g each)
2 rashers back bacon, excess fat trimmed (about 25g each once fat removed)
2 Portobello mushrooms, sliced into 1cm strips
250g asparagus spears
80g spinach or baby spinach, washed
2 large free-range eggs
salt and black pepper

• Preheat the oven to 220°C/200°C fan/gas 7. Lightly grease a large lipped baking tray or roasting tin with half the oil.
• Place the sausages in the tin with the tomatoes and put the tray in the oven. Bake for 10 minutes.
• Take the tray out, turn the sausages and add the bacon, mushrooms and asparagus. Return to the oven for another 5 minutes, or until the sausages and bacon are starting to go golden brown.
• Use the remaining oil to coat the spinach (put it all in a bowl and give it a quick massage). Take the tray out of the oven and clear some space for the eggs. Crack the eggs straight on to the base of the tray, add the spinach and return the tray to the oven for a final 4–6 minutes, or until the eggs are cooked to your liking.
• Season to taste and serve immediately.

MAKE IT VEGGIE: Swap the pork sausages for a vegetarian alternative (but check the labels because they can be salty), scrap the bacon and add another a mushroom and 60g spinach.

ALL-IN-ONE BAKED EGG CUPS

Makes 12 egg cups

These are genius little cupcakes that fill you up and are super-easy to carry around with you if you need to eat your breakfast on the go.

8 large free-range eggs
1 **tbsp** coconut oil
1 red onion, peeled and finely chopped
1 orange pepper, seeds removed, diced
100g broccoli florets, roughly chopped
60g closed cup mushrooms, roughly chopped
60g frozen peas
50g reduced fat Cheddar cheese, finely grated
10g fresh chives, finely chopped
5g fresh parsley, finely chopped
salt and black pepper

- Preheat the oven to 180°C/160°C fan/gas 4 and line a 12-hole muffin tin with paper cases.
- Crack the eggs into a large mixing jug and season to taste. Beat well with a fork and then leave to one side.
- Heat the coconut oil in a large frying pan over a medium heat. Add the onion and pepper and cook for 4–5 minutes, or until they start to soften. Add the broccoli, mushrooms and peas and cook for another 3–4 minutes.
- Stir the cooked veg into the egg with the grated cheese and chopped herbs.
- Divide the mixture between the 12 muffin cases, filling each one to about three quarters of the way. Make sure all the veg is evenly distributed.
- Place into the oven and cook for 18–20 minutes, or until they are golden brown and risen.
- Serve two egg cups per person.

TIP: These are great hot, but are fab for eating cold for breakfast on the go in the week when time is precious! Leave any uneaten egg cups to cool, they will keep in the fridge for three or four days in an airtight container.

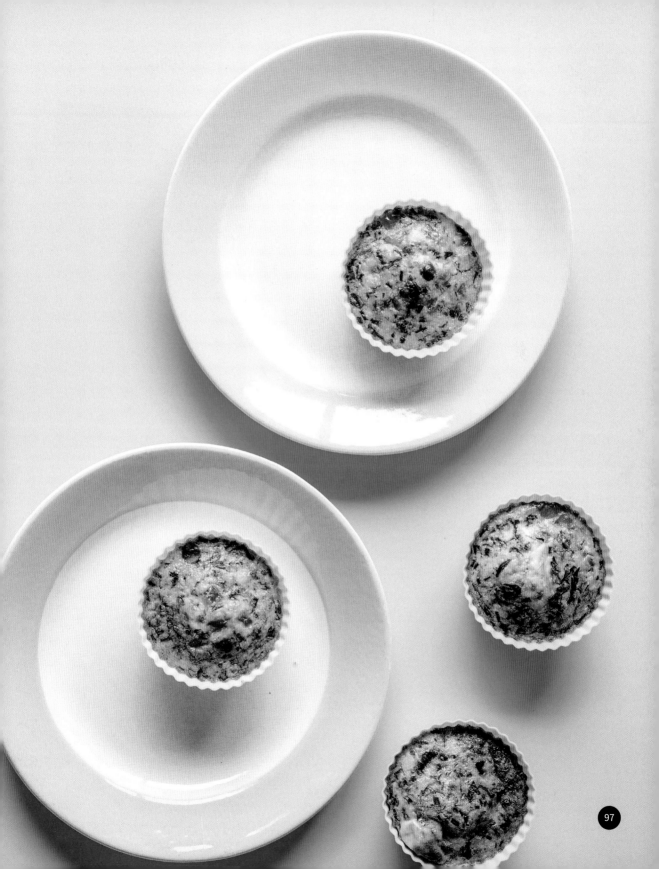

COCONUT PANCAKES WITH MANGO & LIME YOGHURT

Serves 4

Coconut is the secret weapon of athletes because the fats in it rev up your metabolism and keep you going that bit longer. Go coconut!

150g gluten-free
self-raising flour
½ tsp baking powder
50g desiccated coconut,
toasted
2 medium free-range eggs
200ml semi-skimmed milk
120ml 0% fat natural
Greek-style yoghurt
1 lime, zest and juice
1 tbsp coconut oil
160g mango, peeled
and diced
1 red chilli, sliced (optional)

- Put the flour, baking powder and desiccated coconut into a bowl and mix. Make a well in the centre and crack in one of the eggs. Beat well and start to incorporate some of the flour. Add the other egg and mix well. Slowly add the milk, mixing well. Leave to stand for 1–2 minutes.
- Meanwhile, combine the yoghurt and lime juice and zest in a small bowl.
- Heat half the coconut oil in a large frying pan over a medium heat. Drop in 4 tablespoons of the pancake batter to make four pancakes. Try not to move them until the sides start to look like they are drying out and you can see air bubbles forming on the surface of the pancake. Flip the pancakes and cook for another 2–3 minutes. Remove the pancakes from the pan and keep warm while you repeat with the remaining coconut oil and batter.
- Serve two pancakes per person, top with the lime yoghurt and scatter with the mango pieces and chilli, if using.

TIP: You can freeze any uneaten pancakes for another day.

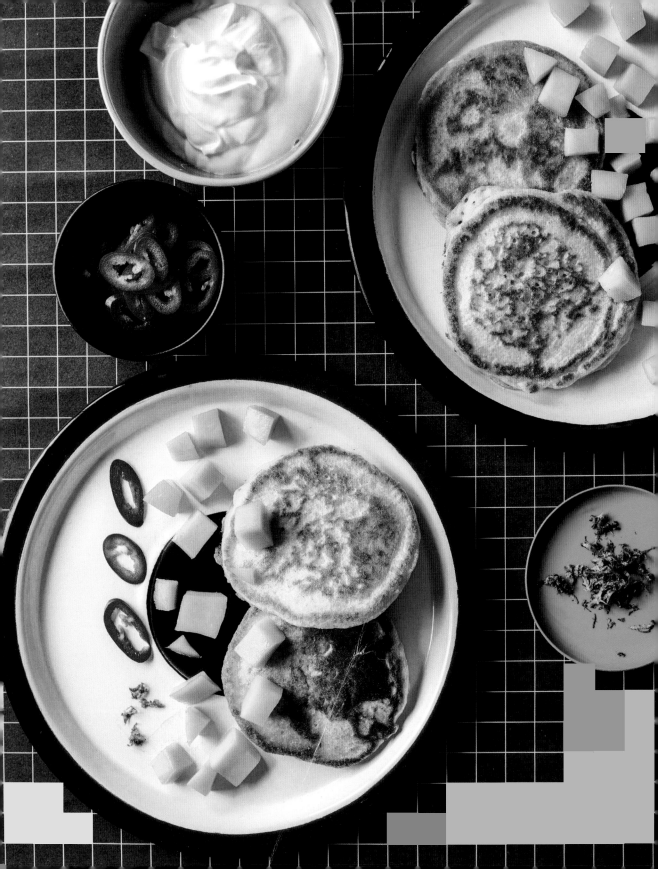

BOILED EGGS WITH RYE CRISPBREAD TOASTS

Serves 2

4 medium free-range eggs,
  room temperature
4 **slices** rye bread
2 **tsp** Sriracha
2 **tbsp** 0% fat natural Greek-
  style yoghurt
1 ripe avocado
a **handful** of cress and/or
  sprouting seeds

Eggs are so talented: they go with so many things! Where would breakfast be without them? And I love some sprouting seeds – they make me feel like a gardener.

- Bring a pan of water to the boil and preheat the grill to high.
- Carefully lower the eggs into the boiling water and cook for 6–9 minutes, depending on whether you want them soft in the centre or not. When the time is up, run the eggs under cold water or they will keep cooking.
- Meanwhile, place the slices of rye bread under the grill. Once they are golden, flip them over to crisp up the other side. Remove to a plate.
- Mix the Sriracha and yoghurt in a dish, and peel and slice the boiled eggs. Cut the avocado in half, remove the stone, peel away the skin and cut into slices.
- To assemble the dish, spread the spiced yoghurt thinly over the four pieces of toast then top with the avocado and finally the egg. Finish with a handful of cress and/or sprouting seeds and tuck in.

TIP: Once you've finished the Blitz you can make a big batch of boiled eggs and keep them in the fridge for snacks or for having this breakfast on repeat – they'll keep for a few days.

BAKED EGG POTS

Serves 2

As I said, eggs are the business in this book and this recipe is no exception. So easy too – just mix it all in a pot and you're done! Egg-stacular!

5g unsalted butter'
240g spinach or baby spinach, washed
16 cherry tomatoes, quartered
150g smoked haddock, flaked
3 tbsp low-fat crème fraîche
2 medium free-range eggs
salt and black pepper

- Preheat the oven to 180°C/160°C fan/gas 4. Lightly grease two 20cm little oven dishes or pie tins with the butter and set aside.
- Heat a large saucepan over a high heat and add a splash of water to make some steam. Tip in the spinach and put the lid on quickly. You want it to start wilting – this should only take 2 minutes.
- Remove the pan from the heat, squeeze the spinach with the back of a wooden spoon and tip out any water. Add the cherry tomatoes, smoked haddock and crème fraîche. Season to taste, mix lightly and divide evenly between the two oven dishes.
- Make a little well in the centre of each dish and crack in an egg. Place the dishes on a baking tray and bake in the oven for 6–10 minutes, depending on how set you like your eggs.
- Remove from the oven and eat straight away.

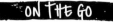
SWEET POTATO MUFFINS

Makes 12 muffins

Ain't muffin wrong with this dish (geddit?!). They're lovely on their own but even better with some nutty spread – you'll be raring to work out!

For the muffins

200g sweet potato, peeled and cut into small chunks
100g carrot, peeled and cut into small chunks
200g gluten-free oats
3 tbsp maple syrup
2 tsp ground cinnamon
200ml semi-skimmed milk
2 medium free-range eggs
100g cashew nut butter
a pinch of salt

For the topping

2 tbsp cashew nut butter
2 tbsp low-fat cream cheese

- Preheat the oven to 180°C/160°C fan/gas 4 and line a 12-hole muffin tin with paper cases.
- Bring a large pan of water to the boil and add the sweet potato and carrot. Cook for 10–12 minutes, or until tender. Drain and transfer to a food processor. Add the oats, maple syrup, cinnamon, milk, eggs, nut butter and salt to the food processor and blitz until everything looks pretty smooth.
- Divide the mixture between the paper cases and cook in the oven for about 25 minutes, or until risen and golden brown. Check they are done by piercing them with a skewer – if it comes out clean they are ready, if not give them another 5 minutes. Cool in the tin for 10 minutes so you can pick them up, then move to a cooling rack. Allow the muffins to cool completely.
- For the topping, mix the nut butter and cream cheese in a small bowl. This mixture will keep in the fridge for 4 or 5 days if stored in an airtight container as will the muffins themselves. Spread a little of it on top of each muffin as you eat them.
- Serve two muffins per person.

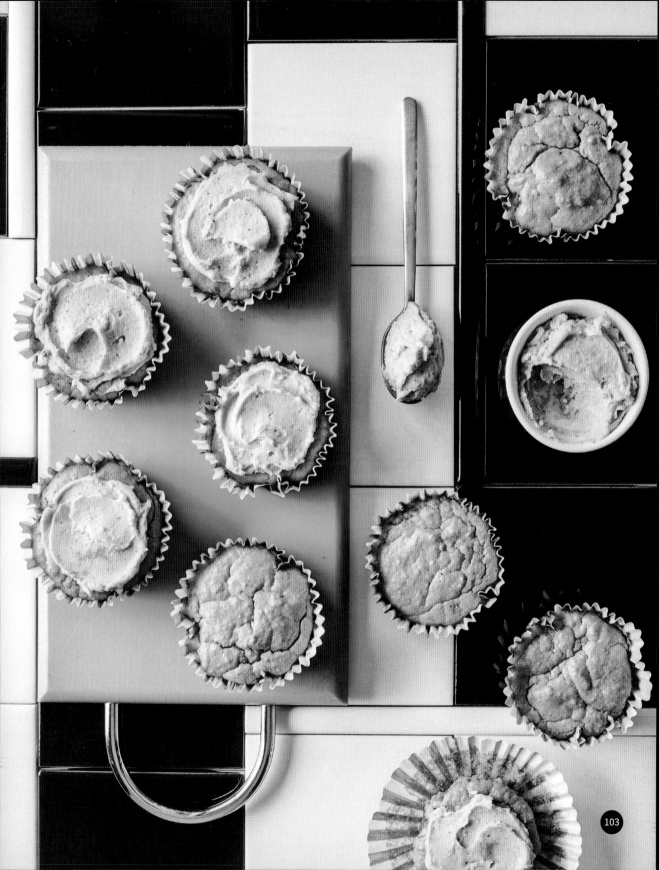

ALMOND & BERRY SMOOTHIE

Serves 2

This is for when you just need to neck something and get on with your day – berry smoothie for a busy bee!

300ml semi-skimmed milk
150g 0% fat natural Greek-
style yoghurt
40g almonds, blanched
160g frozen berries
(make sure there are
lots of blueberries and
raspberries)
1 lemon, zest and juice
a small handful of fresh
berries
a few almond slivers

- Tip all the ingredients, except for the fresh berries and almond slivers, into a blender and blitz for 4–5 minutes until it is really smooth. If it's too thick, just add a little splash of water.
- Serve in large glasses garnished with some fresh berries and almond slivers.

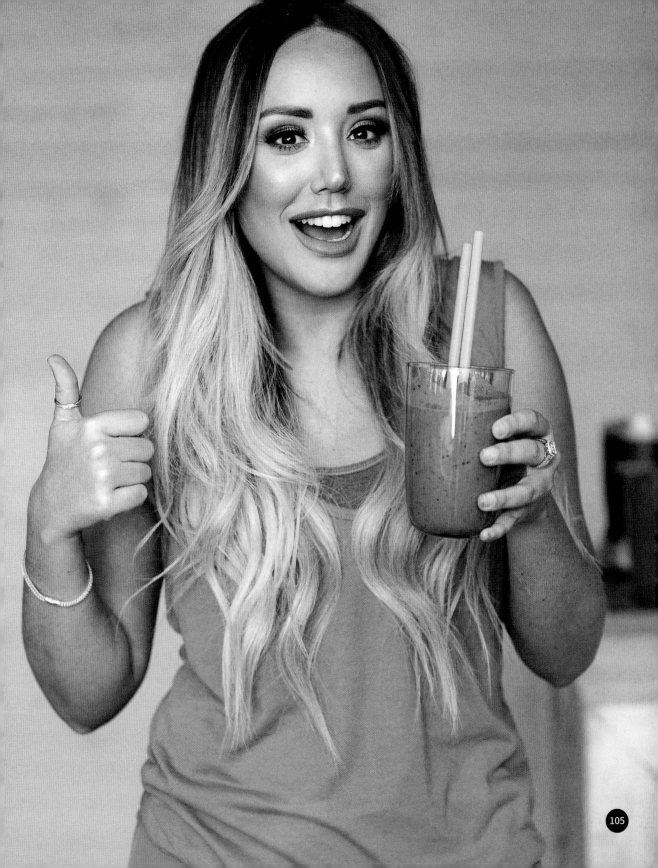

OMELETTE – THREE WAYS

Serves 1

People always say three's a crowd – but not when it comes to omelettes it's not! Three is the magic number (and gives you more choice so you never get bored).

Basic omelette

2 large free-range eggs, beaten well
5g unsalted butter
salt and black pepper

- Crack the eggs into a mixing bowl and beat well with a fork. Season to taste and set aside.
- Heat the butter in a non-stick frying pan over a medium heat. Turn down the heat and pour in the eggs. When the egg starts to set, gently draw it from the edges into the middle of the pan using a heatproof spatula, then tip the frying pan so the uncooked egg fills the gaps. Cook for a further 2–3 minutes or until the mixture is almost set. Turn off the heat, flip one edge of the omelette over and roll or fold it in half. Slide onto a plate and serve.

VEGETABLE OMELETTE

1 small red onion, peeled and finely chopped
30g broccoli, cut into florets and chopped
80g chestnut mushrooms, thinly sliced
7 cherry tomatoes, halved
20g low-fat Cheddar, finely grated
1 red chilli, finely chopped (optional)

- Heat the butter in a non-stick frying pan over a medium heat. Add all the vegetables and cook, stirring every now and again, for 7–8 minutes, or until they have started to soften. Reduce the heat to low, pour in the beaten eggs and cook following the Basic omelette method above.
- Once the omelette is almost set, sprinkle over the Cheddar and chilli, if using. Roll or fold the omelette, slide onto a plate and serve.

PROTEIN PACKED OMELETTE

20g chorizo, finely chopped
80g chard, roughly chopped
1 tbsp cottage cheese
½ tbsp hemp protein powder

- Heat the butter in a non-stick frying pan over a low heat. Add the chorizo and chard and cook gently so the oils from the chorizo slowly start releasing into the pan. Stir every now and again for about 6 minutes.
- Add the cottage cheese to the eggs and mix well. Pour the eggs into the pan and cook following the Basic omelette method. Sprinkle over the protein powder while the egg is still a little bit wet.
- Once the omelette is almost set, roll or fold, slide onto a plate and serve.

MAKE IT VEGGIE: Swap the chorizo for a veggie alternative (but check the label because they can be salty).

MEXICAN OMELETTE

4 spring onions, finely chopped
1 green chilli, finely chopped
60g spinach or baby spinach, washed and roughly chopped
½ tsp smoked paprika
a handful of fresh coriander leaves, chopped
a pinch of chipotle chilli flakes (optional)

- Heat the butter in a non-stick frying pan over a medium heat. Add the spring onions and chilli. Cook, stirring every now and again, for 3–4 minutes, or until they have started to soften. Add the spinach and paprika and cook for another 2 minutes. Reduce the heat to low, pour in the beaten eggs and cook following the Basic omelette method.
- Once the omelette is almost set, sprinkle over the coriander and chilli flakes, if using. Roll or fold the omelette, slide onto a plate and serve.

LUNCH

I used to either eat way too much at lunch and then want to sleep for the rest of the day (carb coma!) or I'd skip it and then want to pig out in the evening. Here's loads of different varieties of lunchtime loveliness so you always have the right balance to your day.

RAINBOW NOODLES WITH SWEET & SPICY SAUCE

Serves 2

Look how colourful this is! In fact, its so bright I think you might need to wear sunglasses while you're eating it.

For the sweet & spicy sauce
1 **tbsp** sriracha
1 **tbsp** mirin
½ **tsp** low-salt soya sauce
½ **tsp** lime juice
½ **tsp** maple syrup

For the noodles
1 **tbsp** rapeseed oil
2 carrots, peeled and spiralised
1 courgette, trimmed and spiralised
1 red pepper, seeds removed, spiralised
1 yellow pepper, seeds removed, spiralised
¼ red cabbage, thinly sliced
¼ white cabbage, thinly sliced
10g fresh coriander leaves, roughly chopped
40g cashew nuts, toasted and roughly chopped
1 **tbsp** sesame seeds, toasted
2 lime wedges

- In a small bowl mix all the sauce ingredients together well.
- Heat the oil in a large wok over a high heat until really hot. Add all the veg and toss quickly in the oil. Cook for 4–5 minutes – you don't want the veg to lose any crunch. Remove from the heat.
- Tip the sauce over the veg noodles and mix really well – you want everything coated in the sauce.
- Divide between two bowls and top with the coriander, toasted cashew nuts and sesame seeds. Serve with lime wedges and hold on tight to your tastebuds!

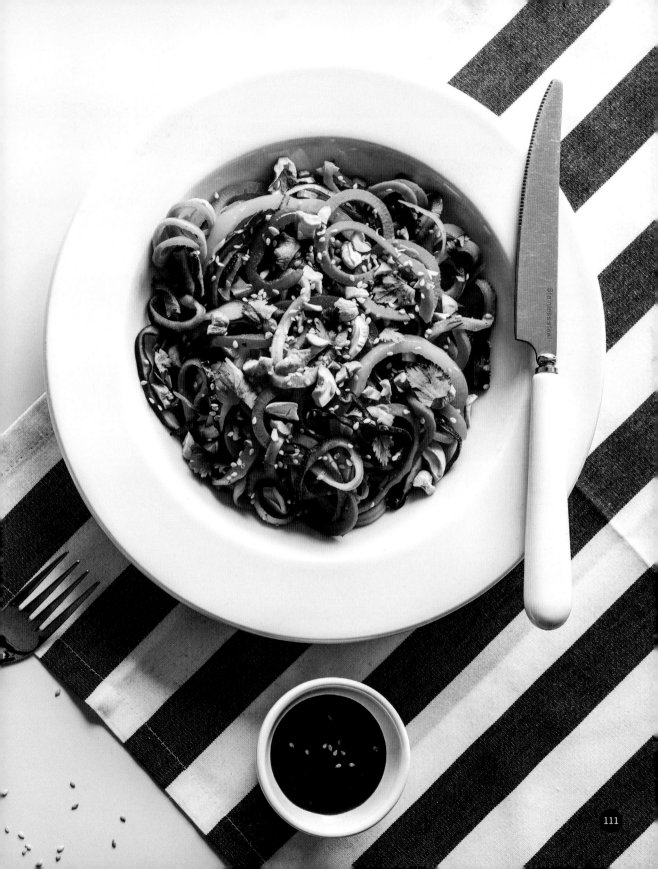

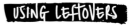

LENTIL RAGU STUFFED PEPPERS

Serves 2

Peppers make the best kind of dishes because you can actually eat them as well as whatever food you stuff inside. Imagine what life would be like if you could always eat the plate as well as the food on top of it! Just don't get so excited about them that you chop the pepper the wrong way (oops!).

1 orange pepper
1 yellow pepper
350g Lentil Ragu with Fresh Tomato Sauce (see page 138)
2 tsp rapeseed oil
120g chestnut mushrooms, sliced
20g hard goats' cheese, finely grated
80g green beans, trimmed
80g Tenderstem broccoli
a handful of fresh basil leaves

• Preheat the oven to 200°C/180°C fan/gas 6 and line a small roasting tin with foil.
• Cut both the peppers in half through the stem. Carefully remove the seeds, trying not to damage the stem or pierce the sides and place the halves in the roasting tin.
• Divide the Lentil Ragu between the four halves.
• Heat the oil in a frying pan over a high heat. When hot, add the mushrooms and toss them quickly for 3 minutes, until they are golden and have lost some of their water. Place on top of the ragu.
• Sprinkle the goats' cheese over the stuffed peppers and cook in the oven for 15 minutes, until the cheese is golden and the peppers have started to soften.
• Meanwhile, bring a large pan of water to the boil and place a steamer over the top. Add the green beans and broccoli and steam for 5–6 minutes, until they have softened but still have a bit of crunch to them. Drain the veg and give them a gentle shake to remove any excess water.
• Remove the peppers from the oven and scatter over the basil leaves. Serve two pepper halves per person with the green veg alongside.

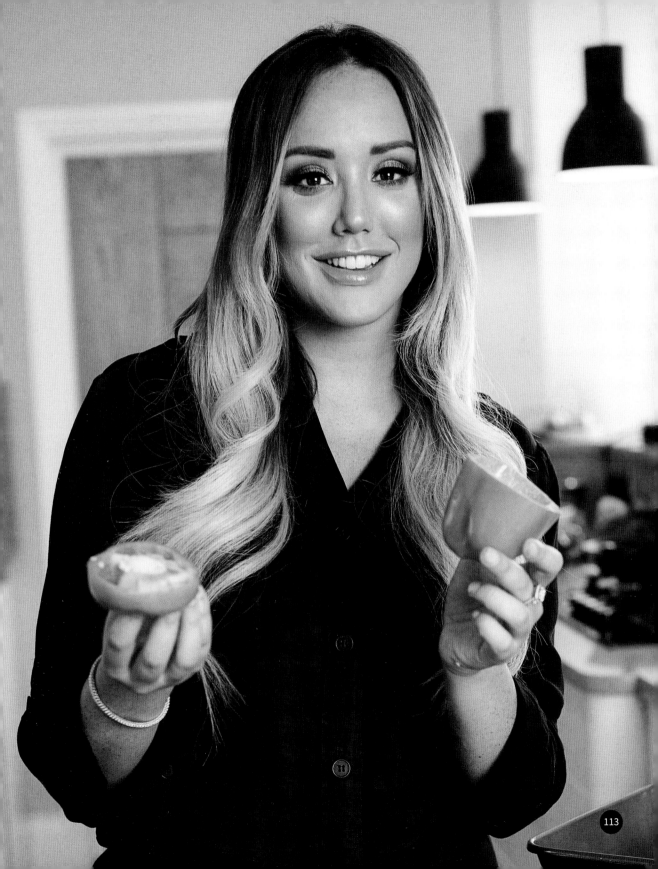

ALL GREEN SOUP

Serves 4

I am a super-fan of soups. They are filling and so good for you – and this one warms you right up just like one of my nan's electric blankets (but not as dangerous).

1 **tsp** olive oil
1 onion, peeled and diced
4 cloves garlic, peeled and finely chopped
1 head broccoli, cut into florets, stalk trimmed and diced (about 450g)
150g spring greens, shredded
100g frozen peas
100g spinach or baby spinach, washed
1 **litre** vegetable stock
½ tsp freshly grated nutmeg
salt and black pepper

- Heat the oil in a large saucepan over a medium heat. Add the onion and cook for 5 minutes, until it has started to soften. Add the garlic and cook for another minute, stirring all the time so it doesn't burn.
- Add the broccoli, spring greens, peas and spinach to the pan, pour in the vegetable stock and bring it to the boil. Reduce the heat and simmer for 12–15 minutes, until all the veg are cooked through and the broccoli stalk is tender.
- Remove the pan from the heat and use a stick blender to blitz it smooth. Add a splash of boiling water if needed until you get the consistency you like. Grate in the nutmeg, season with a little salt and pepper, mix well and serve.

TIP: You can store this in the fridge for a couple of days or freeze it for a couple of months. Serve with a few chilli flakes sprinkled over the top if you like a bit of spice.

GRILLED SALMON WITH ITALIAN COURGETTE SALAD

Serves 2

This takes a bit longer than some of the recipes but it's worth it. Salmon is so good for you I seriously reckon it gives you extra brain cells. And you can use those brain cells to learn to speak Italian because Italy's where your salad comes from.

2 salmon fillets, skin on (about 120g each)
1 tsp runny honey
2 large courgettes, trimmed
2 carrots, peeled
80g rocket
1 tbsp extra-virgin olive oil
1 lemon, zest and juice
½ tsp dried oregano
10g fresh basil leaves
15g pine nuts, toasted
salt and black pepper

- Preheat the grill to its highest setting and line a grill pan with foil.
- Place the salmon fillets on the grill pan, skin side down. Brush the salmon flesh with the honey and pop the tray under the grill for 6–8 minutes, until the salmon caramelises. Remove from the heat and set aside.
- Cut the courgettes and carrots into ribbons using a Y-shaped peeler and place in a large salad bowl. Add the rocket leaves and drizzle over the oil and lemon juice. Sprinkle with the lemon zest and oregano and season to taste. Divide between two plates.
- Using the back of a fork, press down onto the salmon fillets to break them into flakes. Place one on each plate, scatter over the basil leaves and pine nuts and serve.

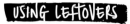

ROAST CHICKEN SALAD
Serves 2

Unless your mam burns the roast chicken (like mine always does) you should be able to keep some of your Sunday dinner and whack it in a salad bowl later in the week.

For the salad
240g ready-cooked skinless chicken (a mix of thigh, leg and breast meat), thinly sliced or shredded
120g mixed lettuce leaves
½ cucumber, sliced into half moons
1 yellow pepper, seeds removed, thinly sliced
12 cherry tomatoes, halved
4 spring onions, sliced on the diagonal
8 radishes, thinly sliced
1 ripe avocado

For the dressing
1 tbsp extra-virgin olive oil
1 tbsp apple cider vinegar
salt and black pepper

- In a large mixing bowl add all the salad ingredients, except for the avocado, and gently toss with your fingers to mix it all together. Divide between two plates.
- Cut the avocado in half, remove the stone then peel away the skin. Cut into slices and top each plate of salad with half an avocado.
- Mix together the dressing ingredients in a small bowl with a little whisk, or use an old lidded jar – just pop everything in and shake it all together.
- Pour the dressing over the salads and enjoy.

TIP: This makes a great packed lunch – just take the dressing with you in Tupperware or an old jar. Pour over just before you eat to keep the lettuce crunchy.

MAKE IT VEGGIE: Replace the chicken with 200g firm pre-cooked tofu, cut into cubes.

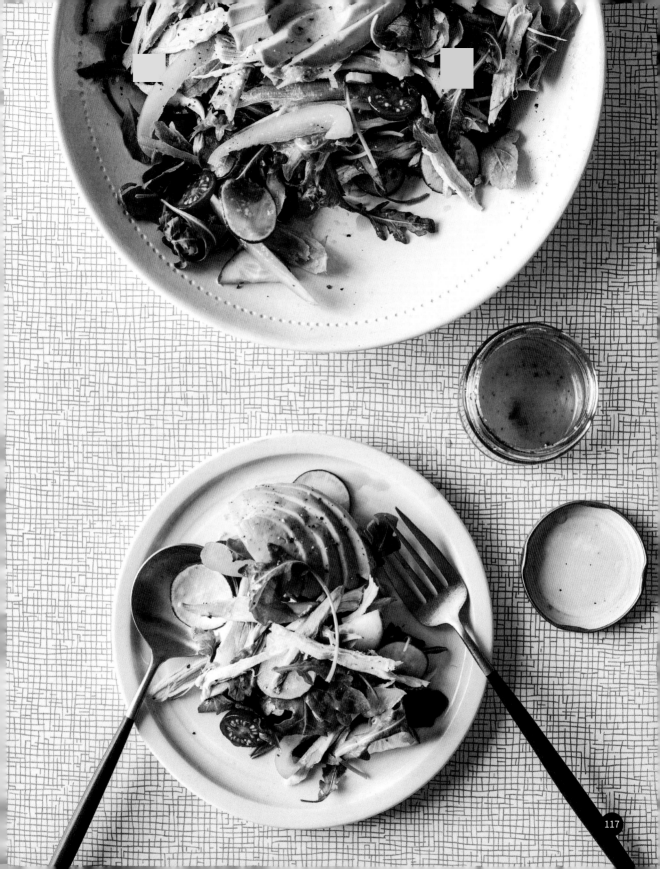

PRAWN COCKTAIL SALAD

Serves 2

Don't get too carried away with the paprika in this recipe because you might end up coughing up the whole thing. Just a sprinkle and the prawns will give you power!

For the salad
1 ripe avocado
120g little gem lettuce, sliced
½ cucumber, sliced into half
　　moons
2 tomatoes, cut into wedges,
　　(about 85g each)
40g radishes, thinly sliced
4 spring onions, thinly sliced

For the prawns
40g low-fat crème fraîche
1 tsp tomato purée
½ tsp Worcestershire sauce
a pinch of ground cinnamon
a pinch of cayenne pepper
200g ready-cooked, peeled
　　king prawns
salt and black pepper

For the garnish
5g fresh chives, finely
　　chopped
a pinch of paprika

• Cut the avocado in half, remove the stone, peel away the skin and cut into chunks. Tip into a mixing bowl and add all the remaining salad ingredients. Toss everything together and divide between two bowls.
• Mix all the ingredients for the prawns – except for the prawns themselves – in a bowl. Season to taste and stir in the prawns to coat them.
• Arrange the prawns on top of the salad, scatter over the chives and garnish with a pinch of paprika.

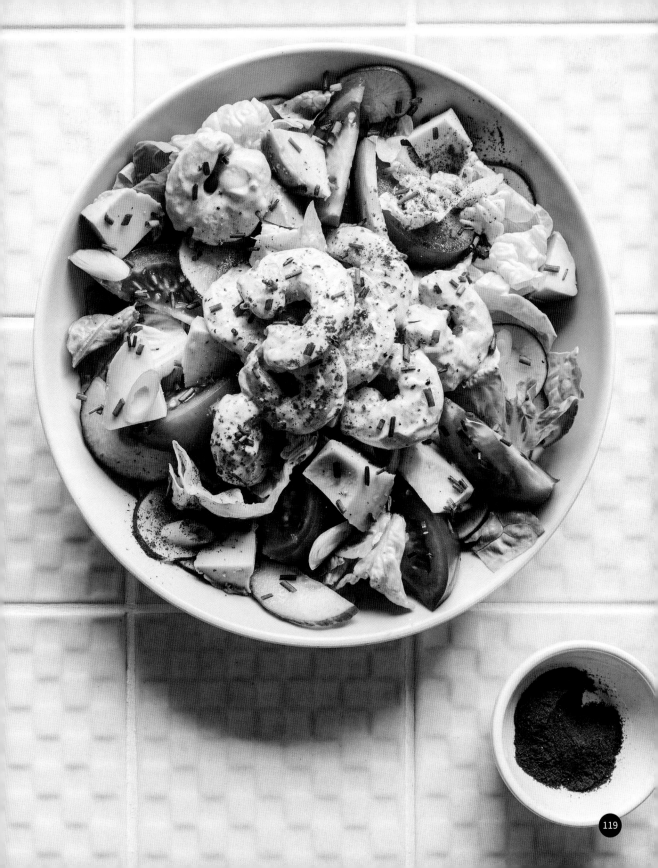

CHICKPEA & JALAPEÑO FRITTERS WITH FETA DIP & ROAST TOMATOES

Serves 3

Don't be fooled by the fact chickpeas have a very strange name (what have they got to do with either chicks or peas?) because they are actually amazingly tasty and good for you. And they go so well with feta which is a cheese you can have on the Blitz.

For the fritters
400g tin chickpeas, drained
100g chickpea/gram flour, plus **2 tbsp** for dusting
3 jalapeños, roughly chopped
2 cloves garlic, peeled and roughly chopped
4 spring onions, roughly chopped
1 **tbsp** paprika
10g fresh coriander, roughly chopped
a splash of milk, if needed
200g cherry tomatoes (on the vine preferably)
2 **tbsp** rapeseed oil
100g green salad leaves
salt and black pepper

For the dip
150ml 0% fat natural Greek-style yoghurt
50g feta, crumbled
1 **tsp** dried oregano
black pepper

- Preheat the oven to 200°C/180°C fan/gas 6 and line a roasting tin with non-stick baking parchment.
- Place the chickpeas, flour, jalapeños, garlic, spring onions and paprika into a food processor and blitz together for a few pulses, until a thick paste is reached – you still want some chunks of everything, though! Tip into a mixing bowl and stir in the coriander, reserving some to garnish, and a little seasoning. If it feels a little crumbly, add a splash of milk. Divide into six patties. Set aside.
- Place the tomatoes on the prepared roasting tin and roast in the oven for 15 minutes.
- Heat the rapeseed oil in a frying pan over a medium heat. Dust the fritters in the extra flour and carefully add them to the pan. Cook for 4–5 minutes on each side until golden and crispy.
- Meanwhile, mix together the ingredients for the dip, adding pepper to taste.
- Serve two fritters per person with the green salad leaves, a dollop of the dip, the reserved coriander leaves and the roasted tomatoes.

TIP: Freeze the leftover fritters – layer between a piece of baking parchment to stop them sticking together – they'll make an easy lunch for one person in the the week after the plan.

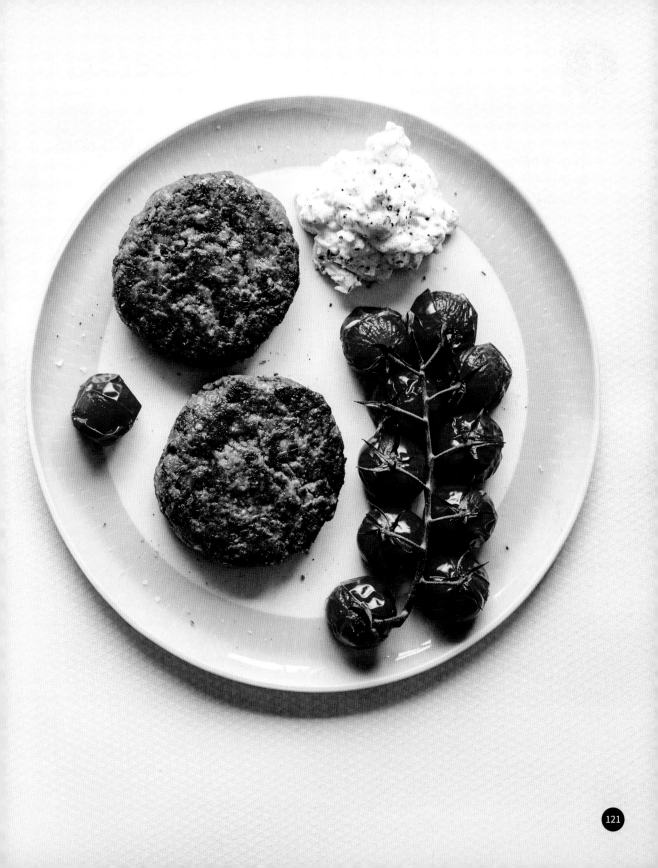

CUCUMBER & MINT SOUP

Serves 2

1 ripe avocado
2 cucumbers, peeled and
seeds removed
160g 0% fat natural Greek-
style yoghurt
1 lemon, juice only
10g fresh mint leaves
salt and black pepper

How delicate and dainty does this soup look? I could stare at this picture forever. I won't though. I will eat it, and so should you.

- Cut the avocado in half, remove the stone then scoop out the flesh with a spoon into a food processor.
- Add all the remaining ingredients with 100ml of water and blitz until really smooth. This will take about 4–5 minutes.
- Season to taste and serve.

TIP: This is a cold soup so all your ingredients need to be really cold before you use them.

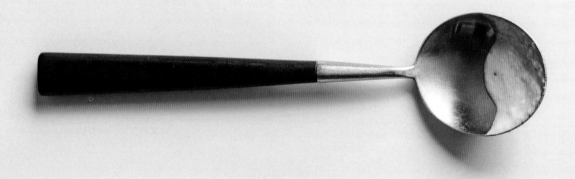

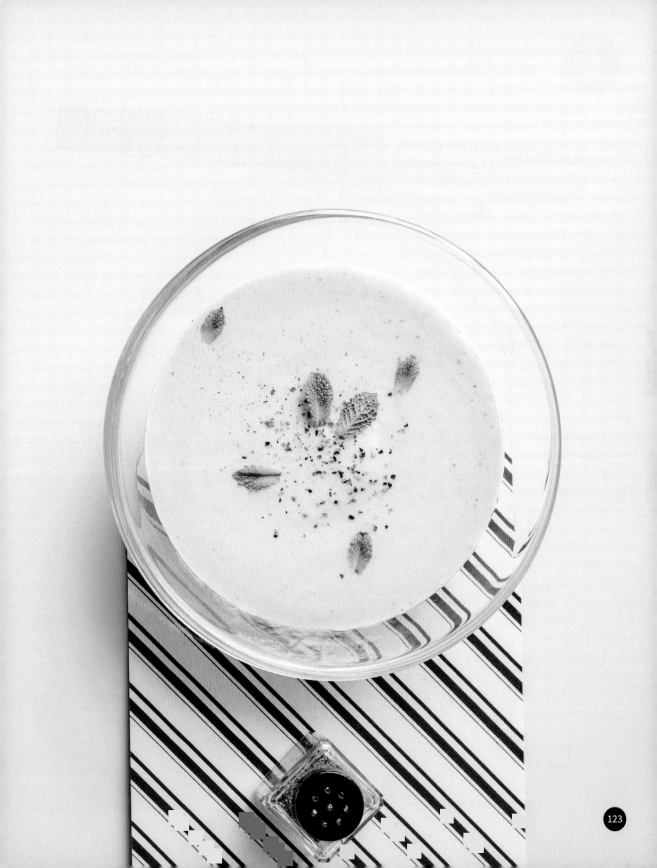

BANG BANG CHICKEN LETTUCE WRAPS

Serves 2

Lettuce is for life, not just for the supermarket. You can use it as a little boat for this chicken and let it sail away down into your stomach.

- 2 boneless and skinless chicken breasts, or 240g ready-cooked skinless chicken, shredded
- **30g** unsalted peanuts
- **1 tbsp** smooth peanut butter (choose one with no added anything)
- **1** small clove garlic, peeled and crushed to a paste
- **½ tbsp** low-salt soya sauce
- **½ tbsp** toasted sesame oil
- **½ tbsp** mirin
- **1** limes, juice only
- **½** cucumber, cut into matchsticks
- **1** large carrot, peeled and cut into matchsticks
- **1** red pepper, seeds removed, thinly sliced
- **1** yellow pepper, seeds removed, thinly sliced
- **4** spring onions, sliced on the diagonal
- **6** cos lettuce leaves
- **2** red chillies, thinly sliced
- **5g** coriander leaves, roughly chopped
- **4** lime wedges, to serve

- Pre-heat the oven to 180°C/160°C fan/gas 4.
- If you are cooking the chicken from scratch, place the two breasts in a deep pan and cover with water. Slowly bring the water to the boil and then simmer for 15 minutes to poach the chicken.
- Place the peanuts onto a baking tray and roast in the oven for 10 minutes, shaking once during the cooking time, until they are a lovely deep golden brown. Transfer to a chopping board to cool and then roughly chop.
- Once the chicken is fully cooked through, remove from the water and allow to cool slightly. Use two forks to pull the chicken into shreds. Set aside.
- Put the peanut butter, garlic, soya sauce, sesame oil, mirin and half the lime juice into a large mixing bowl. Whisk it all together really well – it may look like it's split but keep going, it will all come together.
- Add the shredded chicken to the mixing bowl and coat it well in the peanut sauce.
- In a separate bowl mix together the cucumber, carrot, peppers and spring onions. Squeeze over the remaining lime juice and toss through.
- Divide the peanut chicken between the six lettuce leaves and top with the veg mix and chopped peanuts. Scatter over the chilli slices and coriander leaves and serve with the lime wedges.

MAKE IT VEGGIE: Replace the chicken with 200g pre-cooked tofu, cut into strips.

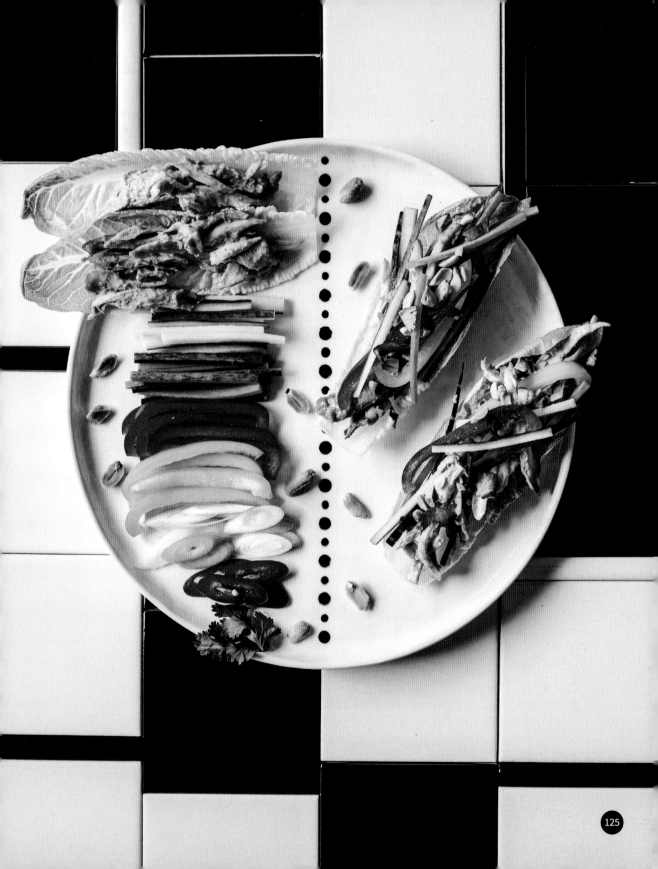

RED LENTIL, PEPPER & CHORIZO SOUP

Serves 4

I love this soup because it's a nice colour and makes you feel all warm inside: red is for romance so maybe have it when you're feeling a bit fruity (or peppery).

200g red lentils
1 tbsp olive oil
1 onion, peeled and finely chopped
2 sticks celery, finely chopped
1 leek, halved lengthways and finely sliced
2 red peppers, seeds removed, diced
3 cloves garlic, peeled and finely chopped
1 red chilli, finely chopped
400g tin chopped tomatoes
1 litre vegetable stock
50g cooking chorizo, roughly chopped
10g flat-leaf parsley, roughly chopped
salt and black pepper

- Rinse the lentils well under cold water.
- Heat the oil in a large saucepan over a medium heat and add the onion, celery, leek and red pepper. Cook gently for 15 minutes, stirring occasionally, until everything is nice and soft. Add the garlic and chilli, stir together and cook for another minute.
- Add the red lentils and mix into all the veg. Stir in the chopped tomatoes, pour in the vegetable stock and bring to the boil. Reduce the heat and simmer for 15–20 minutes, until the lentils are cooked through.
- While the soup is finishing, place a frying pan over a high heat. When really hot, add the chorizo and cook until golden and crispy – this should take about 5–6 minutes. Pour away any oil that comes out of the chorizo while cooking.
- Season the soup to taste and serve topped with the crispy chorizo and a sprinkling of parsley.

TIP: The soup can be stored in an airtight container in the fridge for 4 or 5 days, or in the freezer for 3 months.

MAKE IT VEGGIE: Replace the chorizo with 25g toasted almonds or pine nuts – you'll need your pan on a medium heat only to toast the nuts.

SWEET POTATO, LENTIL & SPINACH SOUP

Serves 4

Sweet potatoes are called sweet for a reason – because they are the prettiest of the potato family and are really good for you. And wouldn't you much rather ask one of them out on a date than an ugly old King Edward?!

200g red split lentils
1 tbsp olive oil
1 onion, peeled and diced
3 cloves garlic, peeled and finely chopped
1cm piece root ginger, peeled and grated
1 green chilli, finely chopped
300g sweet potato, peeled and cut into 1cm dice
1 tsp ground cumin
1 tsp ground coriander
160g baby spinach, washed
salt and black pepper

To garnish
4 tsp low-fat natural yoghurt
a handful of coriander leaves
green chilli slices (optional)

- Rinse the lentils well under cold water.
- Heat the oil in a large saucepan over a medium heat. Add the onion and cook for 5 minutes, until it has started to soften. Add the garlic, ginger and chilli and cook for another minute, stirring all the time so they don't burn. Add the sweet potato and lentils and mix everything together in the pan. Sprinkle in the cumin and coriander and stir to coat all the veg.
- Pour in 1.25 litres of water and bring to the boil. Reduce the heat and simmer until the sweet potato is soft enough to squash with a fork and the lentils are cooked through – this should take 15–20 minutes.
- Remove the pan from the heat and use a stick blender to blitz the soup smooth. Add a splash of boiling water if needed until you get the consistency you like. Return the pan to a low heat and add the spinach. Stir it into the soup until it has just wilted. Season to taste.
- Add a teaspoon of yoghurt to each serving and swirl it through the soup. Top with some fresh coriander and green chilli, if using.

TIP: The soup can be stored in an airtight container in the fridge for 4 or 5 days, or in the freezer for 3 months, so is a great lunch stand-by on a busy morning.

GRILLED CORN, AVOCADO & CHILLI CHICKEN SALAD

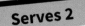
Serves 2

Americans do the best salads and grilled corn is often one of the secret ingredients. The problem is that in America they slather all salads with fatty dressings. But not here, this is super-slimming and good for you.

2 boneless and skinless chicken breasts
½ cauliflower, broken into florets
1 tbsp chipotle chilli paste
2 corn on the cob
120g mixed baby leaves
14 cherry tomatoes, halved
a bunch of spring onions, sliced
1 ripe avocado
5g coriander leaves, roughly chopped
1 lime, cut into wedges

• Preheat the oven to 200°C/180°C fan/gas 6 and line a small roasting tin with non-stick baking parchment.
• Place the chicken breasts and cauliflower in the roasting tin. Spoon over the chipotle paste and rub it all over. Bake in the oven for 20 minutes, or until the chicken is cooked through. Remove from the oven and set aside.
• Meanwhile, bring a large pan of water to the boil and add the corn. Cook for 8 minutes then drain.
• Place a griddle pan over a high heat and char the corn – this will take 10–15 minutes.
• Place the salad leaves, cherry tomatoes, spring onions and roasted cauliflower in a large serving bowl. Cut the avocado in half, remove the stone then peel away the skin. Cut into slices and add to the salad. Pour over any juices from the chicken.
• Using a sharp knife, slice the charred corn kernels from the husks and scatter them over the salad. Finally, slice the chicken breasts into strips and top the salad.
• Serve topped with the coriander leaves and a good squeeze of lime.

MAKE IT VEGGIE: Replace the chicken with 180g aubergine.

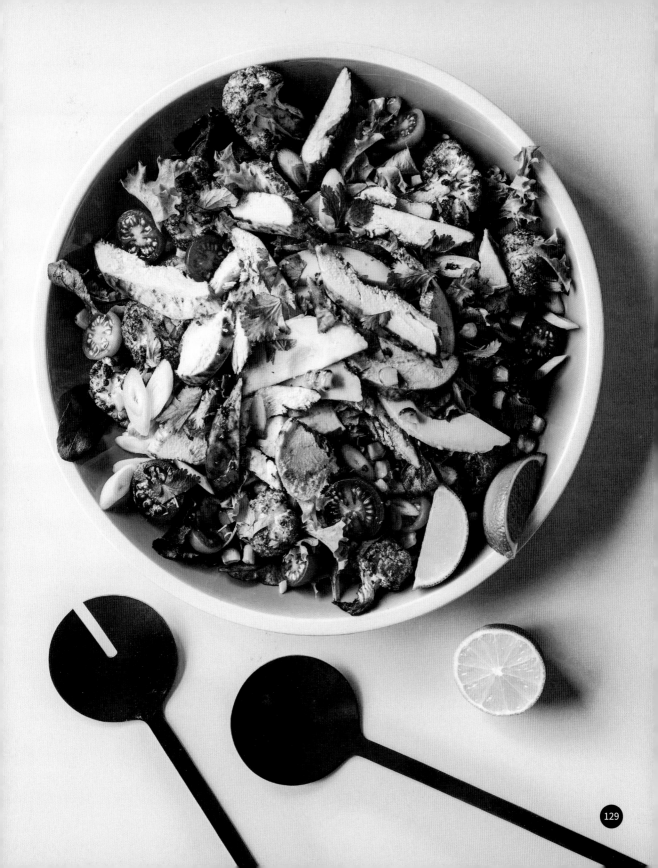

DINNER

Dinner, dinner, you are such a winner. With my recipes you will also be a bit thinner (but not too thin – don't worry, this is a healthy plan!). This section won't make you a sinner – it has such tasty food you won't help but grin(ner).

SWEET POTATO NOODLE PAD THAI

Serves 2

Another genius use of those sweet sweet potatoes: as a substitute for noodles. All the taste and nothing on the waist.

1 **tbsp** rapeseed oil

2 red chillies, finely chopped

1 lemongrass stalk, very finely chopped

25g fresh coriander, roughly chopped

2 **tsp** low-salt soya sauce

2 **tsp** fish sauce

1 **tbsp** oyster sauce

1 medium free-range egg, lightly beaten

a bunch of spring onions, sliced

400g sweet potato, peeled and spiralised

200g beansprouts

1 lime, juice only

40g unsalted peanuts, toasted and roughly chopped

4 lime wedges

• Heat the oil in a wok or large, deep frying pan over a high heat. Add the chilli, lemongrass and coriander, reserving some for garnish, and cook for 2 minutes. Stir in the soya, fish and oyster sauce then the egg, stirring really quickly so it scrambles into the coriander, lemongrass and chilli.

• Add the spring onions, sweet potato noodles and beansprouts and cook, moving everything regularly (tongs can really help here), for 3–4 minutes, until the noodles just start to become tender. Squeeze over the juice from one of the limes.

• Toss in most of the peanuts then divide everything between two bowls. Scatter over the reserved coriander leaves and the remaining nuts and serve with the lime wedges.

TIP: See page 124 for instructions for toasting peanuts.

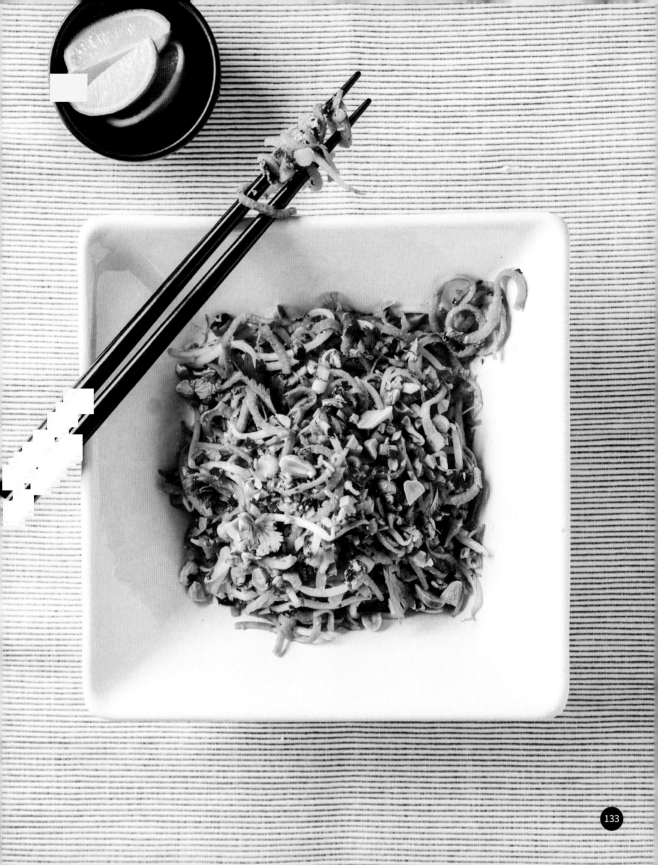

JERK PRAWNS, RICE & PEAS WITH MANGO, PINEAPPLE & CHILLI SALSA

Serves 2

For the brown rice
70g brown rice
100g frozen peas
100g tinned kidney
    beans, rinsed

For the salsa
1 red onion, peeled and
    finely chopped
100g mango, peeled and
    finely chopped
100g pineapple, peeled and
    finely chopped
100g sweetcorn
2 red chillies, finely chopped
5g mint leaves, finely
    chopped
black pepper

For the prawns
1 tbsp rapeseed oil
10g mint leaves
1 onion, peeled and finely
    chopped
3 cloves garlic, peeled and
    finely chopped
2 cm piece root ginger,
    peeled and finely chopped
1 tbsp jerk seasoning
220g raw king prawns
2 lime wedges

I love this meal – not only because the word 'jerk' always makes me laugh, but also because the mango salsa is so yummy I could eat it all day and night (but obviously I won't).

- Cook the rice according to the packet instructions, adding the beans for the last 10 minutes and the peas for the last 5 minutes of the cooking time.
- Meanwhile, assemble the salsa. Put all the ingredients into a mixing bowl and stir together well. Set aside so the flavours start to mingle.
- Heat the oil in a wok or large, deep frying pan over a high heat. Add the mint leaves and cook for 1–2 minutes, until sizzling and crispy. Add the onion, garlic and ginger and cook for another 3–4 minutes, until just starting to turn golden brown. Stir in the jerk seasoning and prawns and cook for a final 3–4 minutes, until the prawns are cooked through. Stir it often to make sure everything cooks evenly.
- Drain the rice of any excess water and serve with the prawns, a good heap of the salsa and a wedge of lime squeezed all over.

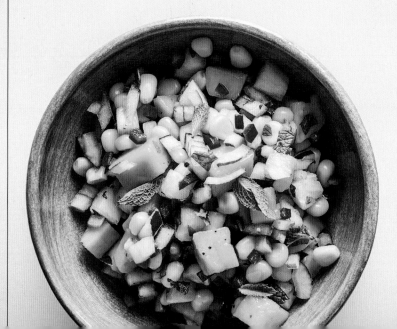

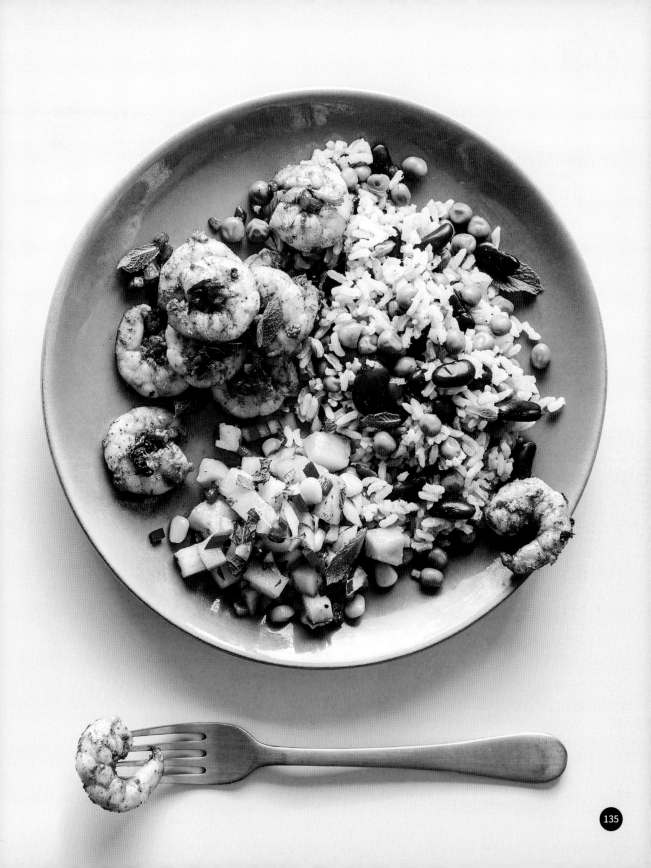

ROASTED SALMON WITH SLAW IN CITRUS DRESSING

Serves 4

For the salmon
500g salmon fillet (in one piece, if possible)
1 **tbsp** runny honey
10g dill, finely chopped

For the slaw
1 red onion, peeled and thinly sliced
½ small red cabbage, thinly sliced
½ small white cabbage, thinly sliced
2 large carrots, peeled and grated
1 fennel bulb, thinly sliced
1 grapefruit, peeled and cut into segments (keep any juice for the dressing)
5g flat-leaf parsley, roughly chopped
5g fresh dill, finely chopped

For the dressing
1 lime, juice and zest
juice from the grapefruit
1 **tbsp** low-fat natural yoghurt
1 **tbsp** olive oil
salt and black pepper

For the veg
200g mangetout
200g sugar snaps, trimmed
200g Tenderstem broccoli

Another salmon meal to make you extra clever. Serve it with my special slaw and you will be so satisfied you'll want to roar!

- Preheat the oven to 220°C/200°C fan/gas 7 and line a roasting tin with non-stick baking parchment.
- Place the salmon in the tin and drizzle over the honey. Sprinkle with the dill and cook in the oven for 15 minutes, until golden brown round the edges.
- While the salmon is roasting, make the slaw by mixing the onion, cabbages, carrots, fennel and grapefruit segments in a bowl. Scatter over the herbs and toss everything together gently.
- In a small bowl mix together the dressing ingredients with some seasoning. Add the dressing to the slaw and gently stir to coat everything.
- When the salmon has 5 minutes left to cook, bring a large pan of water to the boil and place a steamer over the top. Add the veg and steam for 5 minutes until they have softened but still have a bit of crunch to them. Drain the veg and give them a gentle shake to remove any excess water.
- Slice the salmon into four and serve each portion with some slaw and veggies.

TIP: This can be kept overnight in the fridge in an airtight container, so any spare portions can be used for lunch the following day.

CHICKEN NUGGETS & SWEET POTATO CHIPS

Serves 2

One of my biggest weaknesses is chicken nuggets – these ones are really tasty and good for you, so you don't need to feel guilty!

For the chips
300g sweet potato, cut into chips
2 tsp rapeseed oil
1 tsp dried oregano

For the nuggets
2 boneless and skinless chicken breasts, cut into strips
2 tbsp gluten-free flour
1 medium free-range egg, beaten
20g ground almonds
50g panko breadcrumbs
2 tsp smoked paprika

For the slaw
¼ white cabbage, thinly sliced
¼ red cabbage, thinly sliced
2 carrots, peeled and grated
1 tbsp low-fat natural yoghurt
1 tbsp cider vinegar
salt and black pepper

- Preheat the oven to 220°C/200°C fan/gas 7 and line two baking trays with non-stick baking parchment.
- Place the sweet potato chips onto one of the baking trays. Drizzle with the oil and sprinkle over the oregano. Use the parchment to rub the oil and oregano all over the chips. Cook in the oven for 30–35 minutes.
- Meanwhile, prepare the nuggets. Get three shallow bowls: put the flour in one; the egg beaten into another; and add the almonds, panko and paprika to the third. First dust the chicken in the flour, then coat it in egg and then cover with the spicy breadcrumb mix. Place the coated chicken pieces on the second baking tray.
- When the chips have been cooking for 10–15 minutes, place the nuggets in the oven. Bake for 20 minutes, turning both the chicken and chips once during the cooking, until the chicken is cooked through and the crust is golden brown.
- Meanwhile, put all the ingredients for the slaw into a mixing bowl and stir together well.
- Serve the nuggets with the chips and slaw.

MAKE IT VEGGIE: Replace the chicken with 200g firm pre-cooked tofu, cut into strips.

LENTIL RAGU WITH FRESH TOMATO SAUCE & COURGETTI NOODLES

Makes 6 portions

Hey, how ragu? That's something you might want to ask your mates over the dinner table. They will probably think you're strange - but then they will taste this delicious dish and think you're amazing.

250g puy lentils
1 litre vegetable stock
a sprig of fresh rosemary
175g red split lentils
2 tbsp rapeseed oil
1 onion, peeled and diced
2 sticks celery, diced
2 carrots, peeled and diced
1 large red pepper, seeds removed, diced
2 tbsp tomato purée
3 cloves garlic, peeled and finely grated
6 tomatoes, cut into chunks (about 85g each)
150g cherry tomatoes
2 tbsp Worcestershire sauce
1 tbsp dried oregano
10g fresh basil, roughly chopped
½ tsp ground nutmeg
2 courgettes, trimmed and spiralised
salt and black pepper

- Rinse the puy lentils well under cold water.
- Place them in a large saucepan with the vegetable stock and rosemary and bring to the boil. Reduce the heat and simmer for 10 minutes.
- Rinse the red split lentils, add them to the pan and simmer for a further 8 minutes. Drain and rinse under cold water to stop the lentils cooking any further. Set aside.
- Heat one tablespoon of the oil in a large casserole dish over a medium heat and add the onion, celery and carrots. Cook for 5 minutes, until it is all softening and starting to go golden brown. Add the red pepper and cook for another 5 minutes. Add the tomato purée and stir well to coat all the veg. Cook for another minute before adding in the garlic.
- Stir in the drained lentils and mix well. Add both kinds of tomatoes along with the Worcestershire sauce and dried oregano. Cover with a lid and cook over a low heat for 10 minutes, until the tomatoes start bursting.
- Remove the lid, stir well and pour in 200ml of water. Add the basil and nutmeg and season to taste. Cover with the lid again and cook, stirring frequently, until you have a thick ragu and the lentils are fully cooked through. This should take around 20 minutes. Turn off the heat, remove the sprig of rosemary and set aside.
- Heat the remaining tablespoon of oil in a large frying pan or wok over a high heat and add the spiralised courgette. Cook for about 2 minutes. You want it to hold its shape and be a little crunchy.
- Divide the courgetti noodles between two plates and top with a big spoonful of the lentil ragu (about 350g per person).

TIP: Triple the courgetti quantity if there are six people eating, or use the remaining sauce in the Lentil Ragu Stuffed Peppers on page 112 or freeze portions for up to 2 months.

ROAST TURMERIC CAULIFLOWER & LAMB CURRY WITH WILD RICE

Makes 4 portions

You'll be so chuffed once you've made this curry that you'll chuck that Indian takeaway menu in the bin!

1 cauliflower, broken into florets
2 tbsp rapeseed oil
1½ tsp ground turmeric
1 onion, peeled and diced
250g lamb leg, excess fat trimmed, diced
2 tbsp medium curry powder
3 cloves garlic, peeled and finely grated
2cm piece root ginger, peeled and finely grated
400g tin chickpeas, drained
400g tin chopped tomatoes
250ml low-fat coconut milk
70g wild rice
200g spinach or baby spinach, washed
140g sugar snaps

TIP: This makes four portions of lamb curry so double the rice and veg quantity if there are four people eating, or freeze the remaining lamb up to 3 months.

- Preheat the oven to 220°C/200°C fan/gas 7 and line a roasting tin with non-stick baking parchment.
- Add the cauliflower florets and drizzle over 1 tablespoon of the oil. Shake over the turmeric and use the parchment to rub the oil and turmeric all over the cauliflower – be careful as turmeric can stain! Cook in the oven for 15 minutes.
- Heat the remaining tablespoon of oil in an ovenproof casserole over a high heat. Add the onion, lamb and curry powder and mix well. Cook for 10 minutes, stirring regularly.
- Add the cooked cauliflower, along with the garlic and ginger and mix well. Add the chickpeas, chopped tomatoes and coconut milk and stir until well mixed.
- Place the casserole in the oven and turn the temperature down to 170°C/150°C fan/gas 3. Cook for 55 minutes.
- Meanwhile, weigh the rice out into a saucepan and cook according to the packet instructions – this usually takes 40–45 minutes.
- Take the casserole out of the oven and add the spinach. Stir it through and leave it to wilt for 5 minutes.
- Meanwhile bring a large pan of water to the boil and cook the sugar snaps for 5 minutes, or until tender.
- Divide the rice between two plates and top each serving with a quarter of the curry and some sugar snaps on the side.

🌱 **MAKE IT VEGGIE:** Just leave out the lamb!

SHREDDED CHICKEN NOODLE SOUP WITH SWEET POTATO NOODLES

Serves 4

As you can tell by now I love a soup – and this is one of the best because it's got so much going on inside it. It's like the zoo of soups! With sweet potato swirls instead of snakes.

2 boneless and skinless chicken breasts
1 tbsp rapeseed oil
1 red onion, peeled and sliced
2 cloves garlic, peeled and thinly sliced
2cm piece root ginger, peeled and sliced into matchsticks
175g chestnut mushrooms, sliced
100g baby corn
1 litre chicken stock
400g sweet potato, peeled and spiralised
150g spring greens, shredded
a bunch of spring onions, sliced
2 red chillies, sliced
2 tbsp low-salt soya sauce (optional)

- Half-fill a pan with cold water then add the chicken. Put the pan over a medium heat and slowly bring the water to the boil. Turn the heat down and leave to simmer for 15 minutes.
- Heat the oil in a wok or large, deep pan over a high heat. When it is hot, add the onion and cook for 2–3 minutes. Add the garlic and ginger and stir for another minute. Add the mushrooms and baby corn and cook for a further 3 minutes.
- Reduce the heat and pour in the stock. Add the spiralised sweet potato and leave to cook in the broth for 6–8 minutes. Add the spring greens and cook for a further 2–3 minutes, until tender.
- When the chicken is cooked, pull it into shreds using two forks. Add it to the broth and let everything cook together for another minute.
- Divide the soup between four bowls and top each one with some spring onion and chilli. Serve with a dash of soya sauce, if you fancy it.

TIP: The soup can be kept overnight in the fridge in an airtight container for any spare portions to be used the following day.

MAKE IT VEGGIE: Replace the chicken with 200g firm pre-cooked tofu, cut into cubes (not shredded!) and replace the chicken stock with a vegetable stock.

ROAST THAI SALMON WITH STIR-FRIED VEG & RICE NOODLES

Serves 4

I love salmon when it's roasted and it goes really well with these greens. The colours look perfect together too – if it was an outfit you'd get loads of compliments (even if you did smell like fish).

500g salmon fillet (in one piece, if possible)
1 tbsp red Thai curry paste
180g rice noodles
2 tsp toasted sesame oil
180g spring greens, sliced
½ savoy cabbage, shredded
120g pak choi, sliced
1 tsp black sesame seeds

- Preheat the oven to 200°C/180°C fan/gas 6 and line a baking tray with non-stick baking parchment.
- Place the salmon on the baking parchment and rub the red curry paste all over the top of the fish. Roast in the oven for 12–15 minutes.
- Meanwhile, bring a large pan of water to the boil and take off the heat. Add the noodles and leave to soak for 5 minutes, stirring occasionally to break up the block. Drain the noodles and run them under cold water to stop them cooking any further. Leave them to drain while you cook the veg.
- Heat the oil in a wok or large, deep frying pan over a high heat. Add the veg and cook for 3–4 minutes until just cooked. Add the noodles to the pan and mix well.
- Flake the salmon and divide into four portions. Serve a mound of the noodles and veg with the flaked fish and scatter over the sesame seeds.

TIP: The salmon keeps well in the fridge for a quick lunch later in the week.

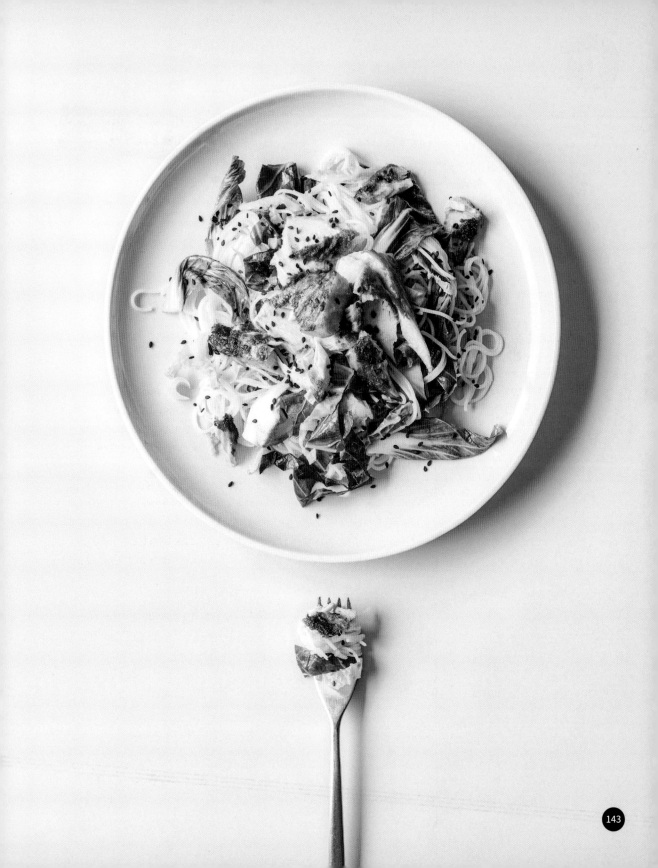

COD TACOS WITH CRÈME FRAÎCHE & GUACAMOLE

Serves 2

I'm sorry but I think this meal looks way too beautiful to eat. So I'm just going to marvel at the colours and lick my lips a lot.

2 cod loins, each weighing around 140g
1 tbsp rapeseed oil
½ tsp smoked paprika
½ tsp garlic powder
½ tsp dried oregano
½ tsp black pepper
½ tsp cayenne pepper
a pinch of salt (optional)
4 corn tortillas
¼ small red cabbage, very thinly sliced
¼ small white cabbage, very thinly sliced
¼ iceberg lettuce, shredded
2 jalapeños, sliced
60g low-fat crème fraîche
4 tbsp Guacamole (2 per servings) (see page 182)
2 lime wedges
a handful of coriander leaves

- Place the cod loins in a shallow dish and drizzle over the oil. Add all the spices and a pinch of salt, if using. Rub the spices all over the fish and set aside to marinate. You can do this the night before, if you prefer.
- Heat a non-stick frying pan over a high heat. Add the fish and cook for 2–3 minutes on each side.
- Meanwhile, warm the four tortillas and place on two plates or a big board. Divide the cabbage, lettuce and jalapeños between the flour tortillas.
- Remove the pan from the heat, flake the cod loins and scatter over the veg.
- Top each tortilla with a dollop of crème fraîche and guacamole, a squeeze of lime and some fresh coriander. Amazing.

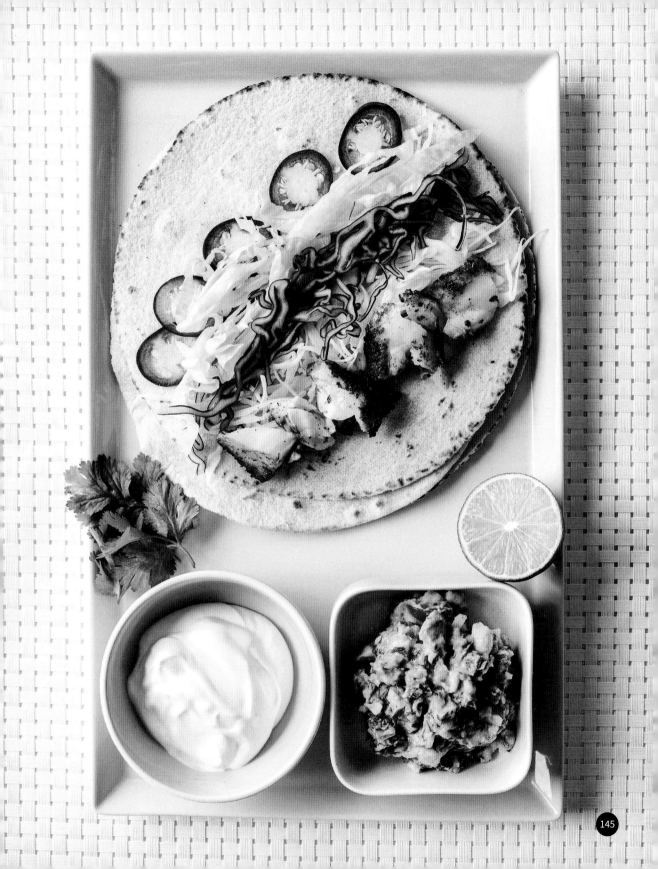

PORK & PEANUT CASSEROLE

Makes 4 portions

1 **tbsp** rapeseed oil
1 onion, peeled and diced
2 cloves garlic, peeled and finely chopped
3cm piece root ginger, peeled and finely chopped
2 **tbsp** tomato purée
1 **tsp** ground cumin
1 **tsp** ground coriander
1 **tsp** cayenne pepper
½ **tsp** ground cinnamon
500g pork shoulder, excess fat trimmed, cut into 3cm pieces
400g tin chopped tomatoes
2 **tbsp** crunchy peanut butter (choose one with no added anything)
2 green peppers, seeds removed, diced
400g tin chickpeas, drained
200g cherry tomatoes
40g unsalted peanuts
300g greens (cabbage/cavalo nero/kale, etc.), shredded
5g fresh coriander, roughly chopped

TIP: The casserole makes four portions so double the quantities of greens if there are four people eating.

I love it when I discover two ingredients that go together. Pork and peanuts are two such things – the perfect match and both begin with P!

- Preheat the oven to 170°C/150°C fan/gas 3.
- Heat the oil in a large ovenproof casserole pot over a medium heat. Add the onion, garlic and ginger and cook for 3 minutes, stirring all the time so nothing burns. Add the tomato purée and coat everything in it. Add all the spices and cook for another minute.
- Add the pork shoulder and coat in the tomato and spices and cook until it changes from pink to white all over – probably about 5 minutes.
- Add the chopped tomatoes, 200ml of water and the peanut butter. Carefully stir until the peanut butter dissolves into the sauce. Turn the heat right down, cover with a lid and simmer for 10 minutes. Once the pork has simmered, cook it in the oven for a further 30 minutes, shaking the tray once during cooking.
- Remove the pot from the oven and stir in the peppers, chickpeas and cherry tomatoes. Return to the oven, without the lid, for another hour.
- Meanwhile, place the peanuts onto a baking tray and place on the bottom shelf of the oven for 10 minutes. Once they are golden brown, remove them from the oven, transfer to a cold plate or bowl and roughly chop when they are cool enough to touch.
- Bring a pan of water to the boil and place a steamer over the top. Add the greens and cook for 4–5 minutes, then drain.
- Give the casserole a good stir and serve portions of the casserole on the steamed greens with a handful of the toasted peanuts and a load of chopped fresh coriander over the top.

MAKE IT VEGGIE: Rather than adapting this recipe for vegetarians I'd suggest having the Butternut Pappardelle instead (see page 166).

WHOLEWHEAT PASTA WITH MIXED VEG SAUCE

Makes 4 portions

Pasta la vista baby! This is a good one if you're a fan of Italian food. It's really filling so will keep you going for hours!

320g wholewheat pasta (penne/fusilli, etc.)

2 tbsp olive oil

1 onion, peeled and diced

1 red pepper, seeds removed, diced

1 yellow pepper, seeds removed, diced

200g cherry tomatoes

1 courgette, trimmed and sliced into half moons

½ head broccoli, cut into florets

a bunch of asparagus, sliced into 4cm pieces

200g chestnut mushrooms, sliced

3 cloves garlic, peeled and sliced

1 tbsp dried oregano

½ tsp grated nutmeg

150g baby spinach, washed

10g fresh basil leaves

20g pine nuts, toasted

20g Parmesan shavings

salt and black pepper

- Bring a large saucepan of water to the boil. Tip the pasta into the boiling water and cook according to the packet instructions.
- Meanwhile, heat the oil in a wok or large, deep frying pan over a medium heat. Add the onion and peppers and cook for 5 minutes. Then add the cherry tomatoes and cook for another 5 minutes. Add the courgette and broccoli and cook for another 5 minutes. The tomatoes should have started to break down by now and will be making a nice sauce to pull everything together. Add the asparagus and mushrooms and cook for 1–2 minutes before adding the garlic and herbs. Simmer everything together for a final few minutes and then stir in the spinach.
- Drain the pasta and add it to the veg. Mix everything together really well.
- Serve the pasta scattered with some fresh basil leaves, toasted pine nuts and a little Parmesan and season to taste.

TIP: Keep any remaining portions in the fridge for lunch the next day.

SEAFOOD PAELLA
Serves 8

Get your mates round and wow them with this amazing feast. It looks like you've been slaving away at the stove all day when you just had to chuck it all in and it was done!

1 **tbsp** rapeseed oil
1 onion, peeled and finely chopped
3 cloves garlic, peeled and finely chopped
2 red peppers, seeds removed, sliced
1 **tbsp** smoked paprika
½ **tbsp** ground cumin
300g brown rice
700ml vegetable stock
200g raw king prawns
300g squid, cleaned
500g clams, cleaned
200g frozen peas
20g flat-leaf parsley, roughly chopped
8 lemon wedges
salt and black pepper

• Heat the oil in a paella pan, or large, deep frying pan, over a medium heat. Add the onion and garlic and cook for 2–3 minutes, stirring to stop them burning. Add the peppers, paprika and cumin and mix well to coat everything. Add the rice and stir gently. Pour in the stock and stir again. Cover with a lid and simmer for 30 minutes.

• Remove the lid, fluff up the rice with a fork and add the seafood, peas and most of the parsley, reserving some to garnish. Mix everything together well, cover with a lid and cook for a further 10 minutes, or until the rice is fully cooked.

• Season to taste and serve with the remaining parsley scattered on top and the lemon wedges on the side.

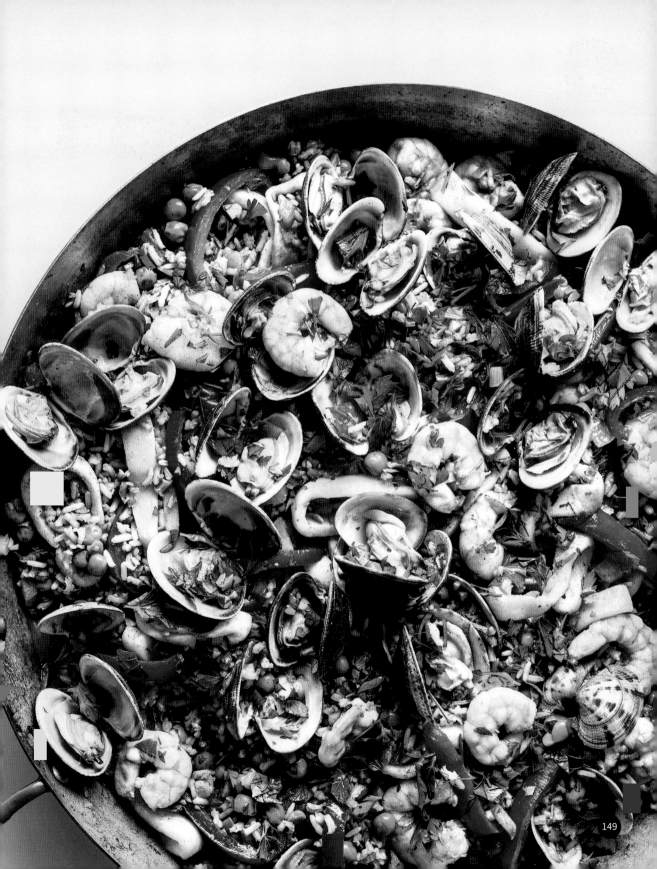

TUNA, BEAN & ROUGH ROMESCO SALAD

Serves 2

Yes I know it looks like I'm randomly carrying round a tray of peppers, but read on… there's a reason and it's called Tuna, Bean & Rough Romesco Salad.

For the salad
1 red pepper
1 yellow pepper
1 orange pepper
3 tomatoes, each cut into 8 wedges (about 85g each)
1 tbsp tomato purée
3 cloves garlic, peeled and sliced
1½ tsp smoked paprika
½ tsp cayenne pepper
1 tbsp olive oil
140g green beans, trimmed and chopped into 3cm pieces
1 courgette, trimmed and sliced on the diagonal into 0.5cm slices
2 tbsp freshly chopped flat-leaf parsley
2 tuna steaks (about 140g each)

For the dressing
1 tbsp extra-virgin olive oil
1 tbsp sherry vinegar or red wine vinegar
salt and black pepper

- Preheat the oven to its highest setting (240°C/220°C fan/gas 9).
- Line a roasting tin with non-stick baking parchment and place the peppers on top whole. Roast in the oven for 30 minutes, turning the peppers once. Remove from the oven and place in a plastic bag and tie the top. Leave them until cool enough to handle.
- Reduce the oven temperature to 180°C/160°C fan/gas 4.
- Throw away the baking parchment and tear the peppers into strips back into the roasting tin, peeling off the skin and discarding the seeds and stalks. Try and catch all the juices. Add the tomatoes, tomato purée, garlic, spices and oil and mix well. Return to the oven for 15 minutes.
- Meanwhile, bring a large pan of water to the boil and place a steamer over the top. Add the green beans and courgette and steam for 5–6 minutes. Drain the veg and give them a gentle shake to remove any excess water.
- Remove the roasting tin from the oven and, using the back of a fork, gently squash everything together. Add the steamed veg to the peppers and tomatoes and scatter with the parsley. Toss everything together and set aside.
- Place a griddle pan over a high heat. When hot, add the tuna steaks and sear for 2 minutes on each side – cook longer if you don't want any pink in the centre.
- To make the dressing, mix the oil and vinegar together with a little seasoning.
- Divide the roast pepper and veggies between two dishes, top with a tuna steak and drizzle over the dressing.

TIP: You could double the quantities of the roast pepper mix to serve later in the week.

VEGETABLE LASAGNE
Makes 6 portions

Lasagnes are usually dripping with oil and fattening sauces but this one replaces béchamel with ricotta, and pasta is swapped for courgette and aubergine. Yum and good for the tum.

2 aubergines, trimmed and thinly sliced lengthways
3 courgettes, trimmed and thinly sliced lengthways
3 **tbsp** rapeseed oil
1 onion, peeled and diced
2 sticks celery, diced
1 carrot, peeled and diced
1 red pepper, seeds removed, diced
1 orange pepper, seeds removed, diced
250g chestnut mushrooms, sliced
3 cloves garlic, peeled and finely grated
1 **tbsp** tomato purée
800g tinned plum tomatoes
2 **tbsp** balsamic vinegar
1 **tbsp** dried oregano
25g fresh basil, roughly chopped
200g ricotta
200ml low-fat natural yoghurt
½ nutmeg, freshly grated
10g Parmesan, grated
salt and black pepper

- Heat a griddle pan over a high heat.
- Brush both sides of the aubergine and courgette slices lightly in 2 tablespoons of the oil. Cook the sliced veg on the griddle pan in batches for 2–3 minutes each side until you have lovely char lines. Remove from the pan and set aside on kitchen paper to absorb any excess oil. Repeat until you have cooked all the slices.
- Heat the remaining tablespoon of oil in a large pan over a medium heat. Add the onion, celery, carrot and peppers and cook for 10 minutes, stirring frequently, until it is all softened and lightly golden brown.
- Add the mushrooms and cook for another minute. Stir in the garlic and tomato purée and mix well. Add the plum tomatoes and break them down carefully with the back of a wooden spoon. Finally stir in the balsamic vinegar, oregano and basil.
- Bring everything to the boil. Reduce the heat and simmer for 30 minutes, stirring occasionally. You don't want it to be watery so if it's still looking a bit thin, keep cooking it a little longer. Season to taste.
- Preheat the oven to 190°C/170°C fan/gas 5.
- While the sauce is cooking, whisk the ricotta and natural yoghurt together in a small bowl and season with the nutmeg.
- When the tomato sauce is thickened, add a third of the sauce to the base of a deep lasagne dish. Cover in a layer of aubergine then a layer of courgette. Add a third of the ricotta mix and spread it out evenly. Top with another layer of tomato sauce, another layer of

aubergine and courgette, and more ricotta sauce. Repeat for a final layer, making sure the ricotta sauce is spread out to cover all the courgette, getting it right up to the edges of the dish.

- Sprinkle over the Parmesan and place on a baking tray in the centre of the oven. Bake for 15 minutes then crank up the heat to 220°C/200°C fan/gas 7 for a final 10 minutes – it should be beautifully golden and bubbly.
- Serve immediately with a green leaf salad.

TIP: You can freeze any leftovers for another day, it will last about 6 weeks.

BLACK RICE NOODLES WITH GREENS & SESAME SEEDS

Serves 2

I love black rice noodles – they look so exotic and cool on your plate. The chilli in this dish really makes it zing – but if you have too much of it your bum will sing!

120g black rice noodles

1 tbsp toasted sesame oil

3 cloves garlic, peeled and sliced

2cm piece root ginger, peeled and finely chopped

140g Tenderstem broccoli, sliced into chunks

100g Brussels sprouts, thinly sliced

100g edamame (soya) beans

100g frozen peas

100g sugar snaps, trimmed and sliced

1 tbsp low-salt soya sauce

4 spring onions, sliced

1 tbsp black sesame seeds

1 tbsp sesame seeds, toasted

1 green chilli, sliced (optional)

a dash of Sriracha (optional)

- Bring a large saucepan of water to the boil. Add the rice noodles and cook according to the packet instructions. Drain in a colander and run under cold water. (You need to stop them cooking or they get really soft and squashy.) Keep them in the colander, draining, while you cook everything else.
- Heat the sesame oil in a large wok or large, deep frying pan over a high heat. Add the garlic, ginger and broccoli stalks – save the florets for later as they don't take as long to cook. Cook for 4–5 minutes, keeping everything moving so nothing burns.
- Add the Tenderstem broccoli, Brussels sprouts, edamame beans, peas and sugar snaps. Cook for 4–5 minutes then add the noodles to heat through. Finally, add the soya sauce and toss it through the noodles.
- Divide between two bowls and top with spring onions, sesame seeds and chilli, if using. If you fancy a really spicy kick, go for a drizzle of Sriracha!

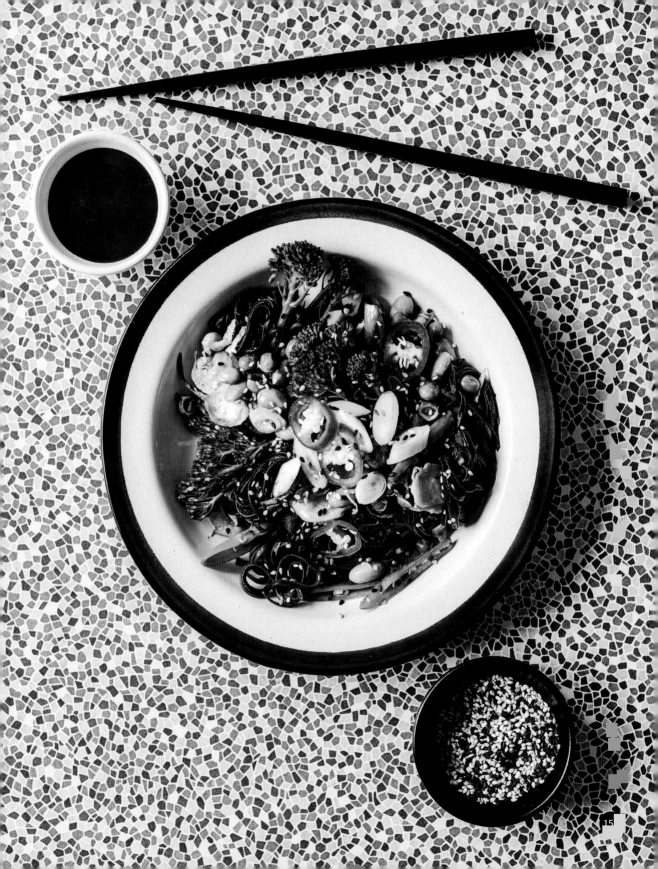

TURKEY CHILLI CON CARNE WITH SHREDDED GREEN VEG

Makes 4 portions

Turkey is the leanest meat you can get and is a great alternative to red meat if you're trying to avoid it like me. This is a lean mean chilli machine.

1 **tbsp** rapeseed oil
1 onion, peeled and diced
1 red pepper, seeds removed, diced
1 orange pepper, seeds removed, diced
2 green chillies, finely chopped
3 cloves garlic, peeled and finely chopped
2 **tbsp** tomato purée
1 **tsp** ground cumin
1 **tsp** smoked paprika
1 **tsp** chipotle chilli flakes
500g minced turkey (5% fat)
400g tin kidney beans, drained and rinsed
400g tin chopped tomatoes
200ml vegetable stock
100g cavolo nero, shredded
100g sweetheart cabbage, shredded
100g spring greens
salt and black pepper

- Heat the oil in a large saucepan over a medium heat and add the onion and peppers. Cook for about 5 minutes. Add the chilli, garlic and tomato purée and mix well to coat everything. Cook for another 30 seconds, then add the spices and the turkey mince. Stir again and break the turkey down. Cook for about 10 minutes, stirring regularly, until the turkey has changed from pink to white-ish.
- Add the kidney beans, chopped tomatoes and stock and stir it all together. Bring to the boil, reduce the heat and leave for about an hour, stirring every now and again. Season to taste.
- About 10 minutes before the turkey con carne is ready, bring a large pan of water to the boil and throw in the greens. Cook for 4 minutes. Drain and divide the veg between two plates. Top each portion with a quarter of the turkey chilli con carne and serve.

TIP: This makes four portions of turkey con carne so double the veg quantity if there are four people eating, or freeze the remaining turkey for another day.

MAKE IT VEGGIE: Replace the turkey with 400g full-flavoured mushrooms (such as portabello), chopped.

CRISPY COCONUT COD WITH PINEAPPLE RICE

Serves 2

I love this dish because (a) the cod tastes lovely all crisped up and (b) pineapple rice is twice as nice (as normal rice).

For the crispy coconut cod
1 tbsp gluten-free plain flour
1 small free-range egg
25g desiccated coconut
40g panko breadcrumbs
400g cod loin
30g gluten-free plain flour or gram flour

For the pineapple rice
70g basmati rice
200g fresh pineapple, diced
1 orange pepper, seeds removed, diced
1 tsp chilli flakes
10g coriander leaves, roughly chopped
2 limes – zest and juice of 1 lime and 1 in wedges

- Preheat the oven to 200°C/180°C fan/gas 6, line a baking tray with non-stick baking parchment and bring a pan of water to the boil.
- Put the plain flour in one bowl, crack the egg in another and beat it lightly, and mix the coconut and panko in a third.
- Dust the cod in the flour, then coat in egg and finally roll it in the coconut breadcrumb mix. Place on the prepared baking tray and cook in the oven for 15 minutes, turning once, until golden and crispy.
- Meanwhile, measure the rice and pineapple into the pan of boiling water and cook according to the rice packet instructions.
- Drain the rice of any excess water and fluff with a fork. Stir in the peppers, chilli flakes and coriander. Squeeze over the lime juice and sprinkle over the zest.
- Serve the cod alongside the pineapple rice. Garnish with more lime wedges, if you fancy.

COURGETTI WITH SPICY CASHEW PESTO

Serves 2

This is such a simple dish and so easy to make especially when you're in a rush or feeling lazy. Cashew pesto is the besto!

For the spicy cashew pesto

70g cashew nuts
2 red chillies, roughly chopped
2 cloves garlic, peeled and roughly chopped
25g basil leaves
30g Parmesan, finely grated
4 tbsp extra-virgin olive oil

For the courgetti

1 tbsp rapeseed oil
3 large courgettes, trimmed and spiralised
5g basil leaves
1 tsp chilli flakes
10g Parmesan shavings
salt and black pepper

- Preheat the oven to 170°C/150°C fan/gas 3.
- Spread the cashews out into a small roasting tin and cook in the oven for 10 minutes, shaking once, or until golden brown all over. Remove from the oven and leave until cool to the touch.
- To make the spicy cashew pesto, blitz the nuts, chilli, garlic and basil in a food processor until you have a smooth paste. Then pulse in the Parmesan and olive oil. Set half of it aside until you need it and put remainder in the fridge for another day.
- Heat the rapeseed oil in a wok or large, deep frying pan over a high heat and add the courgetti. Toss for 2–3 minutes – you want them to hold their shape and not be soft or squashy. Remove from the heat and stir through half the spicy cashew pesto.
- Divide between two bowls and scatter over the basil leaves, some chilli flakes, some Parmesan shavings and a little seasoning. Eat immediately!

TIP: You can keep the pesto for tomorrow's lunch in a small airtight container in the fridge for a week or so and used as a dip with vegetable sticks. Just cover with a little more olive oil to seal it – you will need to throw this away before you use the pesto.

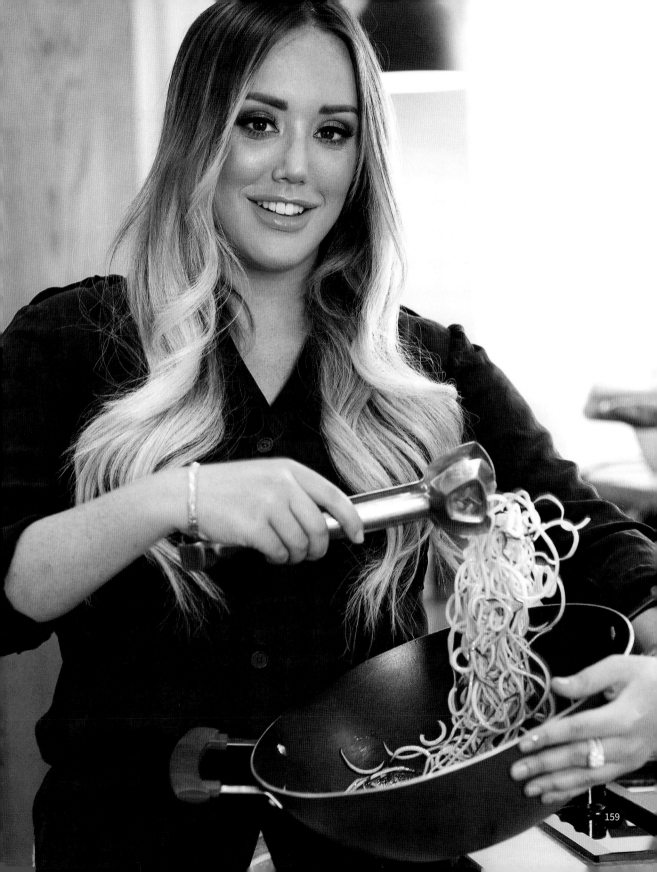

COTTAGE PIE WITH ROOT VEG MASH

Makes 4 portions

Once again sweet potato comes to the rescue and gives you a substitute for creamy mash. This time its joined by Peter Parsnip who adds a whole new twist to this dish!

For the cottage pie
1 tbsp rapeseed oil
1 onion, peeled and roughly chopped
2 carrots, peeled and diced
2 sticks celery, diced
1 green pepper, seeds removed, diced
1 clove garlic, peeled and finely chopped
250g lean minced beef (less than 5% fat if you can get it)
250g ready to eat Puy lentils
350g passata
2 tbsp Worcestershire sauce
salt and black pepper

For the root veg mash
225g parsnips, peeled and cut into 1cm dice
225g sweet potato, peeled and cut into 1cm dice

For the green veg
½ savoy cabbage, shredded
200g mangetout
200g peas

- Preheat the oven to 200°C/180°C fan/gas 6.
- Heat the oil in a large saucepan over a medium heat. Add the onion and cook for 5 minutes until it starts to soften. Add the carrots, celery and pepper and cook for another 5 minutes. Add the garlic and stir for 30 seconds before adding the beef. Continue to cook until the mince has browned. Add the lentils, passata, Worcestershire sauce and season a little. Leave this to simmer for 30 minutes.
- Meanwhile, place the parsnips and sweet potato in another saucepan and cover with cold water. Bring to the boil and cook for 15 minutes or until tender. Drain the water and mash the veg together. It should have enough moisture in it to make a good smooth mash. Set aside.
- Place the mince in the base of a deep 28cm oven dish and level the top. Cover with the root veg mash and cook in the oven for 20–25 minutes.
- Meanwhile, bring a large pan of water to the boil and place a steamer over the top. Steam the cabbage, mangetout and peas for 5 minutes. Drain and set aside.
- Put half the pie to one side for another day, then divide the remainder and the veg between two plates.

TIP: The pie makes four portions so simply double the quantities of veg if there are four people eating. Otherwise, enjoy the leftover pie for a lunch in the week or freeze for another dinner. It will last 3 months.

MAKE IT VEGGIE: Replace the mince with another 250g pouch of Puy lentils.

GARLIC CHILLI PRAWNS WITH WILD RICE & GREEN BEANS

Serves 2

I always wonder what makes rice 'wild'. Does it mean it likes going out on the town? If so, this is the sort of rice I like. Me and wild rice are destined to be best mates.

100g wild rice
140g green beans, trimmed
140g mangetout
2 tbsp rapeseed oil
4 cloves garlic, peeled and thinly sliced
2 red chillies, thinly sliced
300g raw king prawns
10g flat-leaf parsley, roughly chopped
2 lemon wedges
salt and black pepper

- Cook the rice according to the packet instructions. Drain the rice of any excess water and keep covered in the saucepan.
- Ten minutes before the rice is due to be ready, bring a small pan of water to the boil and add the veg. Cook for 4–5 minutes, then drain and keep warm while you cook the prawns.
- Heat the oil in a wok or large, deep frying pan over a high heat. When hot, add the garlic, chilli and prawns all at once. Stir-fry very quickly for 4–5 minutes, until the garlic is really fragrant and the prawns are cooked through. Season to taste.
- Stir the parsley through the wild rice and divide between two bowls. Top with half the prawns and drizzle over any cooking juices. Serve alongside the veg with the lemon wedges and eat straight away.

CRISPY CHILLI BEEF STIR FRY WITH LOADS OF VEGGIES

Serves 2

I love stir fries and Chinese food – this is one for all you meat lovers out there.

1 tbsp cornflour
1 tsp five-spice powder
200g lean steak (frying steak/ bavette/rump, etc.), excess fat trimmed, cut into thin strips
2 tbsp rapeseed oil
1 red onion, peeled and sliced
3 cloves garlic, peeled and finely chopped
3cm piece root ginger, peeled and finely chopped
2 red chillies, finely chopped
½ broccoli, cut into small florets
120g baby corn
120g mangetout
½ savoy cabbage, shredded
salt and black pepper

- In a mixing bowl stir together the cornflour, five-spice and some salt and pepper to taste. Add the strips of beef and toss in the spiced flour to coat well.
- Heat 1 tablespoon of the oil in a large wok or large, deep frying pan over a high heat and add the onion, garlic and ginger. Toss in the hot oil for a minute before adding the chilli, broccoli, baby corn and mangetout. Stir-fry for 4–5 minutes before adding the cabbage. Cook for another 3–4 minutes.
- Transfer the veg to a bowl and heat the remaining oil in the pan over a high heat. Add the beef and cook for 1–2 minutes, depending on whether you like it medium or well-done, before returning the veg to the pan to heat through.
- Serve on two big plates.

MAKE IT VEGGIE: Replace the beef with 100g full-flavoured mushrooms (such as portabello) and two colourful peppers, sliced.

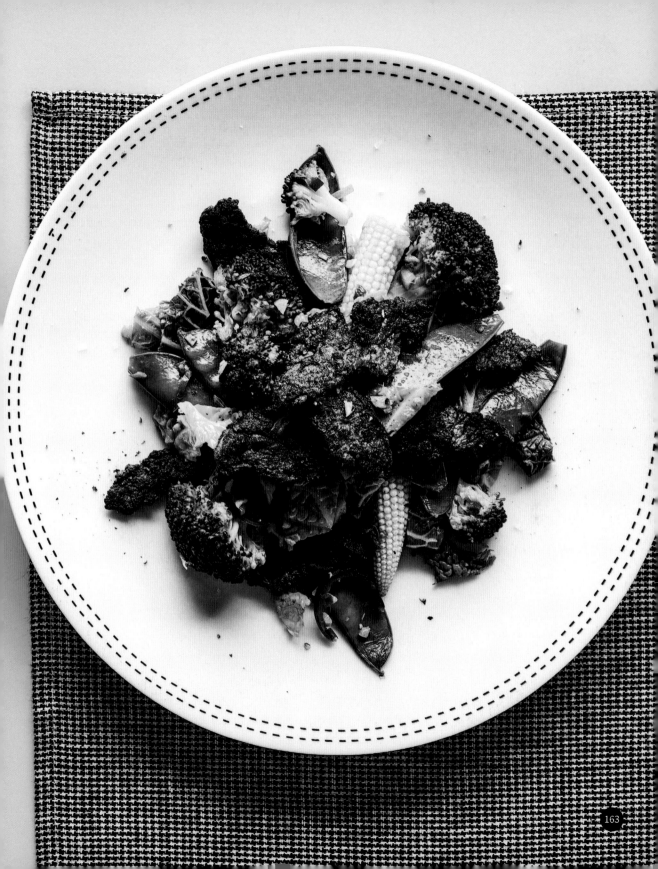

ROAST CHICKEN, ROAST VEG & STEAMED GREENS

Makes 4–6 portions

I know I always go on about how much I love a roast, but I really do. Even me mam's – if it doesn't go too wrong. And the great thing about the roast chicken in this plan is that it gives you lots of leftovers for some easy lunches later in the week.

For the roast chicken

1 free-range chicken, approx. 1.8–2kg
10g fresh sage leaves
2 bay leaves
3 cloves garlic, peeled and left whole
2 tsp olive oil
1 tsp smoked paprika
1 tsp dried sage
1 tsp cumin
salt and black pepper

For the roast veg

¼ butternut squash, peeled and cut into chunks
2 parsnips, peeled and cut into chunks
6 cauliflower florets
6 baby leeks
1 tbsp rapeseed oil
salt and black pepper

Cont…

- Preheat the oven to 220°C/200°C fan/gas 7 and line a roasting tin with non-stick baking parchment.
- Place the chicken in the tin and put the sage leaves, bay leaves and garlic cloves into the cavity. Drizzle the olive oil over the bird, making sure you get the breasts, thighs and legs. Sprinkle with the paprika, dried sage and cumin and a little seasoning, if you like, and make sure to rub it all over. Roast the chicken on the middle shelf of the oven for 70 minutes.
- Meanwhile, place the veggies for roasting in a large roasting tin in a single layer. Pour over the rapeseed oil and mix the veg well with your hands to coat them. Season the veg and place on the bottom shelf of the oven for the last 30 minutes of chicken's cooking time.
- Remove the chicken from the oven and cover with a piece of non-stick baking parchment and a clean towel. Allow it to rest for at least 10 minutes – this will make it extra juicy when you come to eat it.
- Meanwhile, give the roasted vegetables a quick stir and move them to the middle shelf and increase the temperature to 240°C/220°C fan/gas 9. Continue to roast the veg while the chicken rests.
- Bring a saucepan of lightly salted water to the boil and drop in the greens. Cook for around 5 minutes, then drain. Put a lid on the pan to keep them warm while you make the gravy.

For the greens
50g cavalo nero, kale or
savoy cabbage, shredded
50g sweetheart cabbage or
spring greens, shredded

For the gravy
300ml fresh chicken stock
2 tbsp cornflour
1 tsp dried sage

- Stir 3 tablespoons of the stock into the cornflour in a small saucepan to make a paste. Place over a medium heat and slowly add the rest of the stock, whisking the whole time. Bring to the boil until it thickens. The cornflour will initially make it cloudy but it will go clear as it continues to cook.
- Carve the chicken and serve about 150g per person, using a mix of breast and leg meat. Split the roasted veg between the two plates and serve alongside the greens and gravy.

TIP: The chicken will serve 4–6 so double the quantities of veg, greens and gravy if there are four people eating. Otherwise, use the leftover chicken for the Roast Chicken Salad on page 116 or Bang Bang Chicken Lettuce Wraps on page 124.

MAKE IT VEGGIE: It's hard to make a vegetarian version of a roast chicken! So when you're doing the plan have Crispy Cod with Pineapple (see page 157) instead.

BUTTERNUT SQUASH PAPPARDELLE WITH RICOTTA, SAGE & PINE NUTS

Serves 2

Yes I know what you're thinking: 'WTF is pappardelle?' Well, it's Italian for 'broad ribbons' so now you know. These ribbons are made from butternut squash – trust me, you'll love them.

1 small butternut squash, peeled (about 400g)
2 tbsp olive oil
10g sage leaves
2 cloves garlic, peeled and finely grated
80g soft ricotta
20g pine nuts, toasted
10g Parmesan, shavings
salt and black pepper

- Start by making the butternut squash pappardelle. Use a peeler to make long, wide ribbons of squash.
- Bring a large pan of water to the boil and place a steamer over the top. Add the squash pappardelle and steam for 3 minutes. Check to see if it's nearly soft and, if necessary, cook for another minute at a time until tender. Drain and set aside.
- Heat the oil in a large wok or large, deep frying pan over a medium heat. Add the sage leaves and let them crackle and crisp for 1–2 minutes. Remove them from the pan using a slotted spoon and drain on kitchen paper.
- Add the squash pappardelle to the pan and turn it over in the oil to make sure it's all coated. Add the garlic and cook for 2 minutes.
- Divide the squash between two bowls and dot with the ricotta. Scatter over the pine nuts and sage leaves and season to taste. Finally, top with the Parmesan shavings and serve.

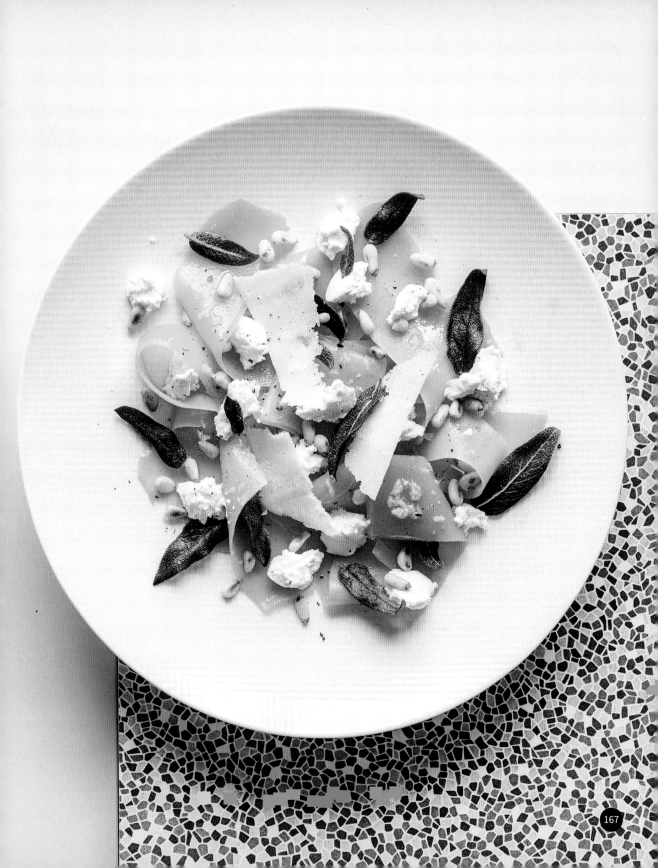

PUDDING

Now this is what I'm talking about. Say the word fast and it sounds like you're a microwave going off: 'Pud-Ding!'

- Knock knock.
  Who's there?
- Pudding.
  Pudding who?
- Pudding your trousers on before your knickers is a silly idea.

BERRY FROZEN YOGHURT

Serves 8–10

Now doesn't this look lovely? I could literally wear this yoghurt as eyeshadow! I won't though because it will melt all over my eyes. And it tastes so divine you'll never want ice cream again.

500ml low-fat natural yoghurt (Skyr is really good for this)
200g frozen berry mix
1 tsp vanilla extract

- Place everything into a food processor and blitz until it is really smooth.
- Transfer to an airtight container and place in the freezer overnight to set.
- Serve a couple of scoops per person.

TIP: If you want it super, super smooth you could sieve it…

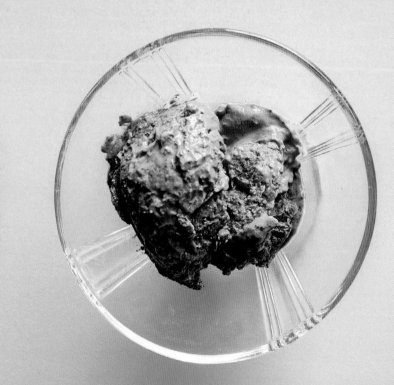

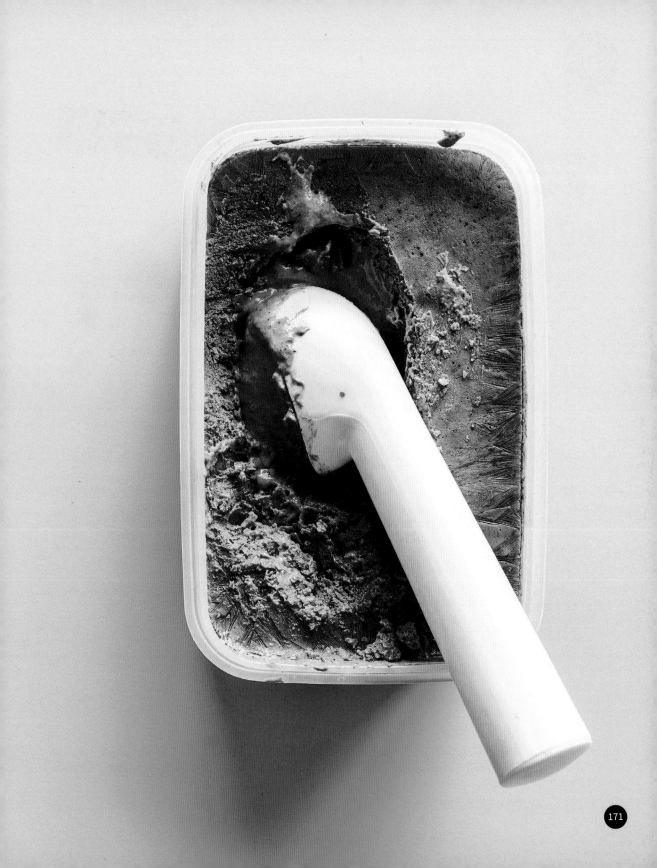

POACHED PEARS WITH VANILLA YOGHURT

Serves 2

Believe it or not it's not just eggs that can be poached. And I don't mean stealing them either.

4 tbsp maple syrup
2.5cm piece root ginger, peeled and sliced
2 ripe but firm Conference pears, peeled but kept whole with stalks intact
120g low-fat natural yoghurt
½ tsp vanilla bean paste

- Place the syrup and ginger into a medium saucepan with 1 litre of water and bring to the boil. Immediately reduce the heat to hold it at a simmer.
- Add the pears to the pan and gently poach them for 20–25 minutes. If they are small pears you may want to reduce the time by a couple of minutes, or if they're bigger you could add on another 5 minutes.
- Mix the yoghurt and vanilla paste together in a small bowl.
- Once the pears are poached, discard the poaching liquid and serve one pear per person with a good dollop of the vanilla yoghurt mixture.

TIP: The maple syrup is just used to flavour the poaching liquid so don't worry if it seems a lot!

CHOCOLATE BOMBS

Makes 10

25g almonds
25g cashews
150g Medjool dates, pitted
1 **tbsp** almond nut butter
1 **tbsp** hemp protein powder
1 **tbsp** raw cacao
½ **tsp** vanilla extract
20g desiccated coconut

You can give these to someone you fancy and say, 'Want a date?' You won't be lying because there *are* dates inside!

- Place both types of nuts into the small bowl of a food processor and blitz until they are crumbs. Add all the remaining ingredients, except for the desiccated coconut. Pulse it a few times to roughly break it down. Scrape down the sides and then let the motor run for 1–2 minutes, until it all comes together.
- Take small spoonfuls of the mixture and roll it into balls with your hands – you want them to be about the size of a ping pong ball and you should make ten.
- Put the desiccated coconut into a shallow bowl or on non-stick baking parchment and roll the balls in the desiccated coconut.
- Serve one chocolate bomb per person.

TIP: Store these in an airtight container for up to two weeks (if they last that long!).

BAKED APPLE & BLACKBERRY WITH MAPLE SYRUP YOGHURT

Serves 2

I love crumble and this tastes just like it.

2 Granny Smith apples,
   peeled, cored and
   quartered
60g frozen blackberries
1½ tbsp maple syrup
120g 0% fat natural Greek-
   style yoghurt
30g pecan nuts

- Preheat the oven to 180°C/160°C fan/gas 4.
- Take a large sheet of foil and fold it in half. Make a little tray out of it by pulling up all the sides.
- Place the apple quarters onto the foil and top with the frozen berries. Pour over the maple syrup and close the foil up into a tight parcel.
- Place the parcel onto a baking tray and cook in the oven for 25–30 minutes.
- Carefully open the parcel, as it will be full of steam, and pour all the juices into a mixing bowl. Add the yoghurt to this liquid and swirl through.
- Serve four quarters of apple per person with half the berries. Crumble over some of the pecan nuts for a bit of crunch and add a dollop of yoghurt.

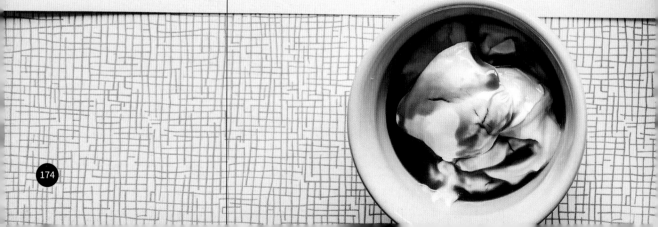

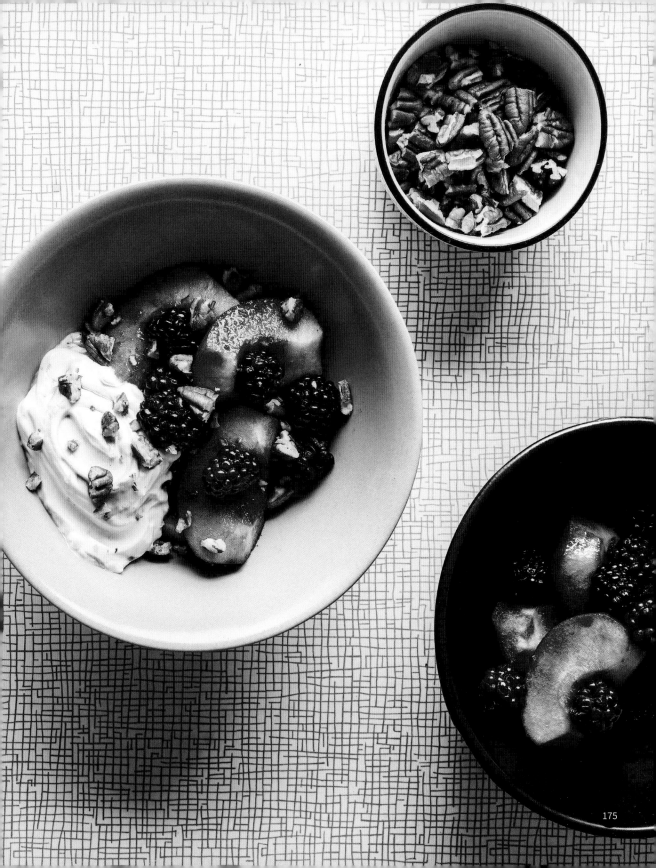

SNACKS

Snacks are very important because if you don't have them you can get very angry (or snackry as I like to call it). Always make sure you have healthy things to nibble on otherwise you might slip up and find yourself swimming in a giant bag of crisps.

VEGETABLE CRISPS

Serves 6

Vegetable… isn't that a weird word? I wonder what it has to do with 'table'? Nothing probably so just eat all these crispy ones and forget I ever mentioned it.

2 parsnips, washed and thinly sliced

2 large sweet potato, washed thinly sliced into rounds

2 large beetroot, peeled and thinly sliced into rounds

150g kale leaves, thick stem removed

1 tbsp olive oil

salt and black pepper

- Preheat the oven to 150°C/130°C fan/gas 2.
- Place all the veg in a large mixing bowl, drizzle over the oil and season to taste. Using your hands, mix the veg and oil together really well.
- Lay out all the veg on two baking trays, trying not to let them overlap too much.
- Place the trays in the oven and roast gently for 30 minutes.
- Remove from the oven, turn the crisps over and return to the oven for another 30 minutes.
- Turn and check again. Pick out any that are done and set aside. Return the remaining crisps to the oven and repeat until they are all crisp and crunchy.

TIP: You could also try flavouring the crisps. For a BBQ flavour, add ½ teaspoon each of ground cumin and sweet smoked paprika; or for something with a kick, try adding 1 teaspoon of chilli powder.

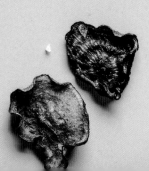

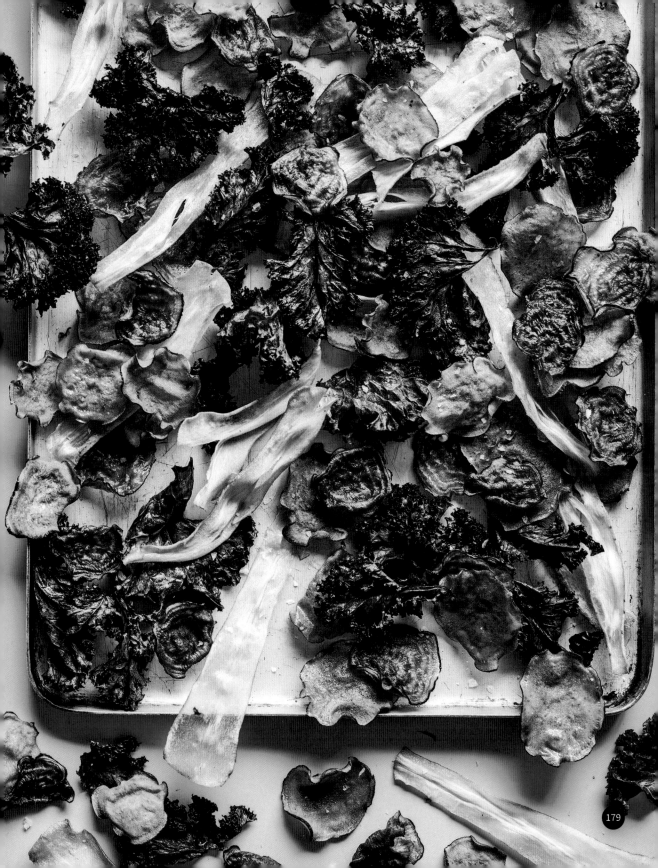

HUMMUS – THREE WAYS

Makes 4–6 portions

Hummus is a very special creation. I don't think there's anything else like it in the universe. It must be good because there's even a restaurant in London called Hummus Brothers. (I'd quite like to meet the owners… just to see what a hummus brother looks like.)

Basic hummus

400g tin chickpeas, well drained
1 clove garlic, peeled and roughly chopped
2 tbsp tahini
1 tbsp olive oil
1 lemon, juice only
½ tsp ground cumin
salt and black pepper

- Place all the ingredients in a food processor with 1 tablespoon of water and roughly pulse everything together. Scrape down the sides and then let the motor run for around 3–4 minutes to make a smooth hummus. You can add 1–2 teaspoons more water if you like it thinner and run the engine again.

ROAST RED PEPPER HUMMUS

150g ready-roasted jarred red
peppers, ideally in brine, drained
1 tbsp sweet smoked paprika

- As per the Basic hummus but add the
peppers and paprika when blitzing.

HERBY LEMON HUMMUS

1 extra lemon, juice only
10g flat-leaf parsley, finely chopped
10g fresh coriander, finely chopped

- As per the Basic hummus but instead of the
juice of 1 lemon, use 2 lemons and leave
out the water. Once everything is blitzed,
stir through the chopped herbs. You could
also use the zest from one of the lemons, if
you want that extra citrus kick.

JALAPEÑO HUMMUS

2 jalapeños, sliced in half, deseeded
(optional) and cut into chunks
1 tsp chipotle chilli flakes

- As per the Basic hummus but add the
jalapeños when blitzing. Scatter over the
chipotle chilli flakes when serving for extra
chilli flavour.

GUACAMOLE & VEG STICKS

Serves 4

What do you call an avocado that's been blessed by the pope? Holy Guacamole!

2 carrots, peeled and cut into batons
2 sticks celery, cut into batons
½ cucumber, cut into wedges
1 yellow pepper, seeds removed, sliced

For the guacamole
2 ripe avocadoes
1 lime, juice only
1 tomato, seeds removed, finely chopped
1 banana shallot, peeled and finely chopped
1 red chilli, finely chopped
10g fresh coriander, roughly chopped
salt and black pepper

- Cut the avocado in half, remove the stone then scoop out the flesh into a mixing bowl. Using the back of a fork, gently mash to break it down. Add the lime juice to stop it browning and mix with the fork.
- Add the rest of the guacamole ingredients and mix well. Season to taste.
- Dunk the veg sticks and enjoy.

TIP: Make a full batch of the guacamole for the Cod Tacos on page 144, for example, and keep the remaining portions for a scrummy snack – store it in a small airtight container. Press a piece of cling film down all over the surface of the guacamole. You want to try and stop any air coming into contact with the avocado, or it may go brown. Place a lid on the container and keep in the fridge for two to three days.

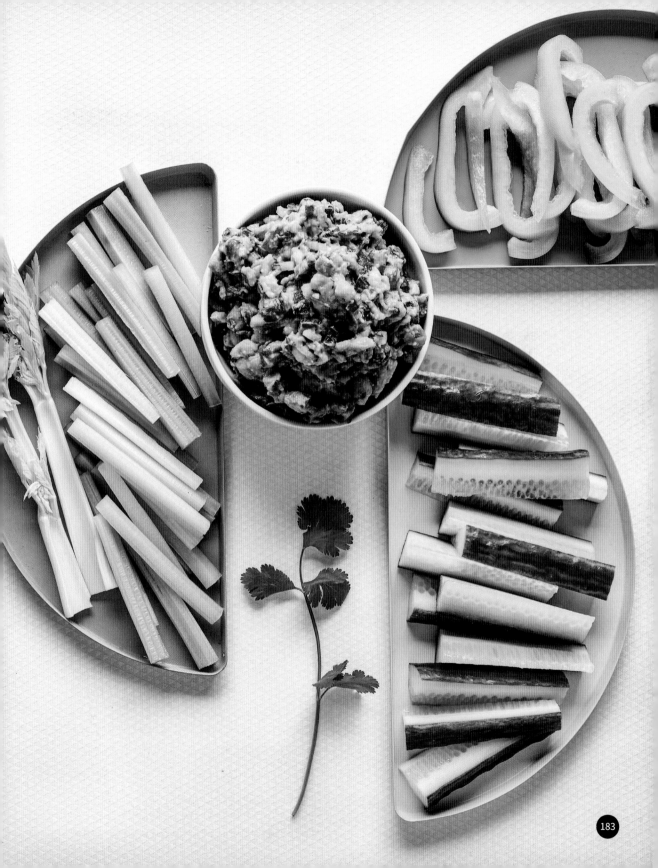

SMOKED TROUT PÂTÉ WITH VEG STICKS

Serves 4–6

Anyone who tells me on social media that I have a trout pout – this one's for you! It's proof that a trout can be delicious and is even better when you dip something in it (like a veg stick in this case).

Ingredients

2 carrots, peeled and cut into batons
2 sticks celery, cut into batons
½ cucumber, cut into wedges
1 green pepper, seeds removed, sliced

For the smoked trout pâté

250g smoked trout
80g low-fat crème fraîche
3 tbsp low-fat natural yoghurt
15g fresh chives, finely chopped
1 lemon, juice and zest
salt and black pepper

- Place the smoked trout, crème fraîche and yoghurt in a food processor and blitz everything together until smooth. Add the chives and lemon zest and mix well. Add the lemon juice a teaspoon at a time until it's zingy enough for you and season to taste.
- Keep chilled until you need it and serve with a heap of the veggies to dip in.

PROTEIN BALLS

Makes 6

I want to write a rude joke here about balls but it's too obvious and the book editor will cut it out. But you know what I mean!

40g ground almonds
60g dates, destoned
25g almond or hazelnut nut butter
20g hemp protein powder
10g coconut oil, melted and cooled
½ tsp ground cinnamon
20g sesame seeds

- Place everything, except the sesame seeds, into the small bowl of a food processor and blitz until well mixed.
- Once the mixture has started coming together, transfer to a mixing bowl and use your hands to bring it all together.
- Shape it into bite-sized balls with your hands – you should make six.
- Place the sesame seeds into a shallow bowl and roll the balls in the sesame seeds.
- Serve one per person.

TIP: Store them in an airtight container for up to 2 weeks.

SPICED NUTS

Makes 12 portions

Please see my earlier comment about protein balls! Nonetheless this is another extremely tasty snack.

1 medium free-range
   egg white
300g mixed nuts – to include
   almonds, walnuts, cashews
   and pecans
½ tsp cayenne pepper
½ tsp hot smoked paprika
¼ tsp ground cumin
¼ tsp ground black pepper

• Preheat the oven to 150°C/130°C fan/gas 2 and line a roasting tin with non-stick baking parchment.
• Lightly whisk the egg white in a mixing bowl until it starts to go white and foamy.
• Tip in the nuts and spices and mix everything together really well until it's all coated.
• Turn the bowl out onto the prepared tray and spread out the nuts. Place the tray in the oven and bake for 10 minutes.
• Remove the tray from the oven and, using a spoon, turn the nuts over and move the ones on the edge into the centre and vice versa. Return the tray to the oven for another 10 minutes, until the nuts are a lovely deep golden colour and super crunchy.
• Allow the nuts to cool completely in the tin before serving in 25g portions.

TIP: Transfer any uneaten nuts to an airtight container. They should stay crunchy for a couple of weeks.

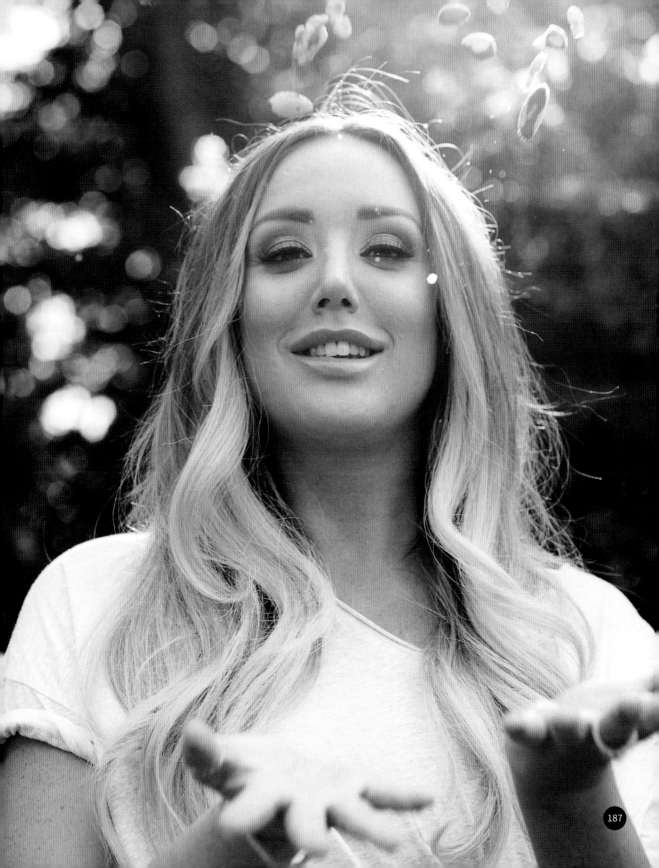

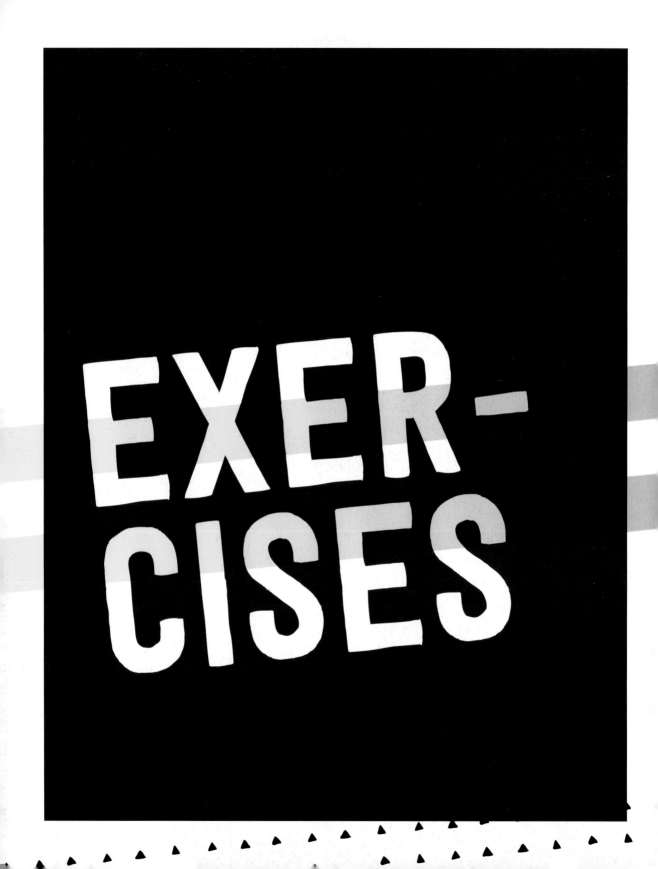

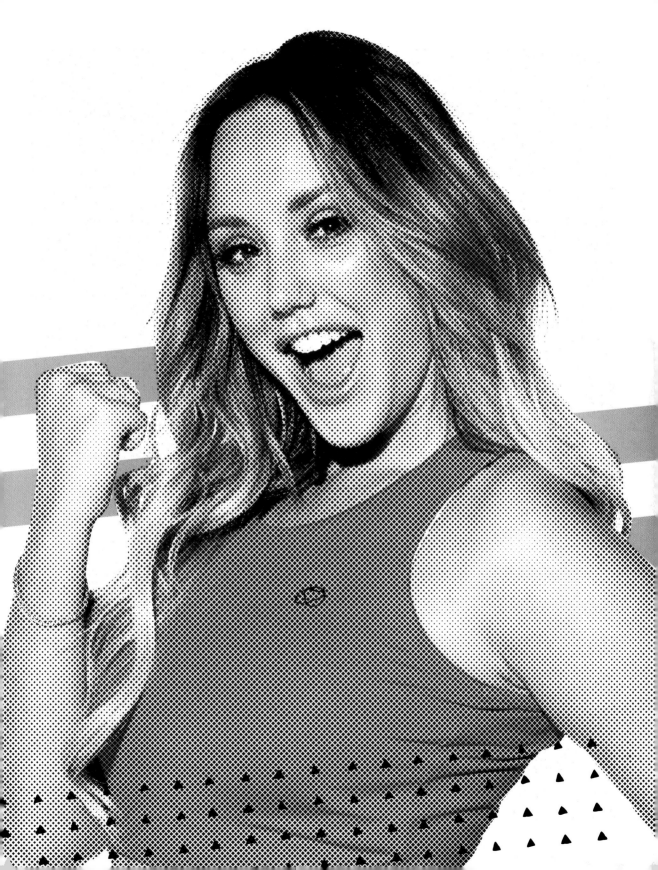

WARM -UP

This quick, effective warm-up will get the blood flowing and mobilise your body so it's prepared for the workout. Aim for 12 to 16 repetitions on each exercise.

* VERTICAL SWINGS

Link hands and bend legs, keeping back straight then swing arms up and bend behind head.

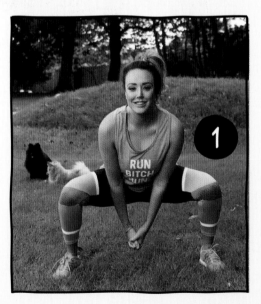

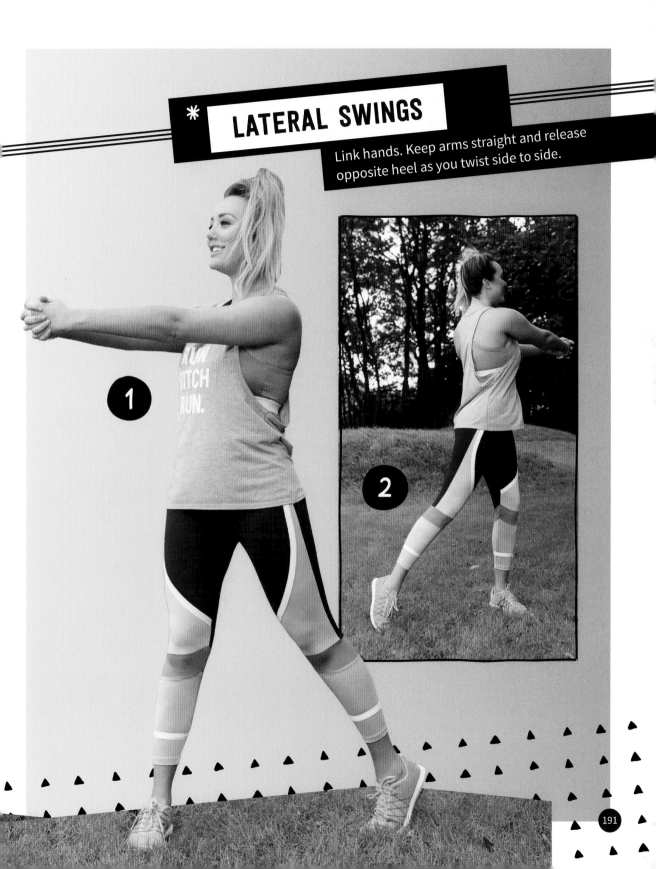

* LATERAL SWINGS

Link hands. Keep arms straight and release opposite heel as you twist side to side.

CONT...

* ALTERNATE LUNGE & REACH

Take a big step forward and push weight through your front heel. Don't let the front knee go over the foot. Focus on the back knee going down. Repeat with the opposite leg.

* BUTT KICKERS

Place your hands on your bum, palms out. Flick your heels into your hands or as high as possible. Take them fast for a high-impact warm-up, or slow for a lower impact.

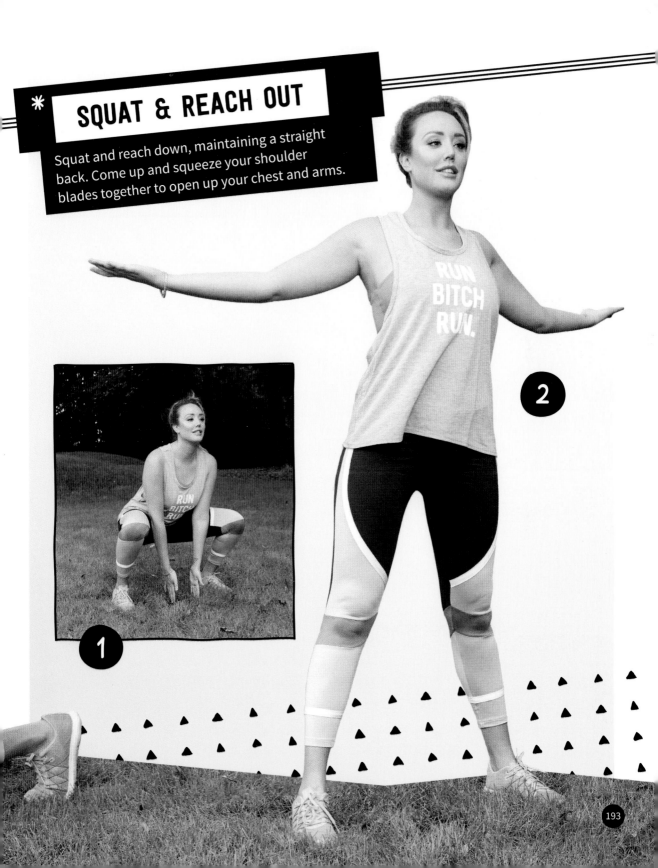

SQUAT & REACH OUT

Squat and reach down, maintaining a straight back. Come up and squeeze your shoulder blades together to open up your chest and arms.

1

2

✳ SPIDY STEP & REACH

This full-body exercise is a great mobiliser.

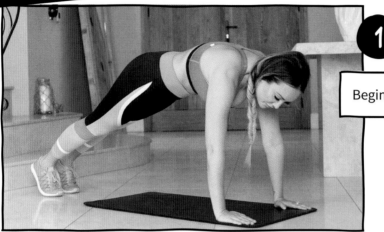

1

Begin in a press-up position. »

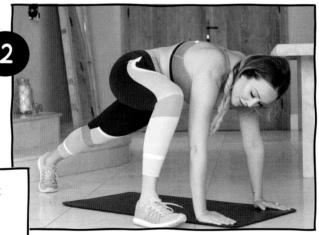

2

Step your right foot forward and to the side (aim for the outside of the right hand). Make sure your heel is flat to the floor. »

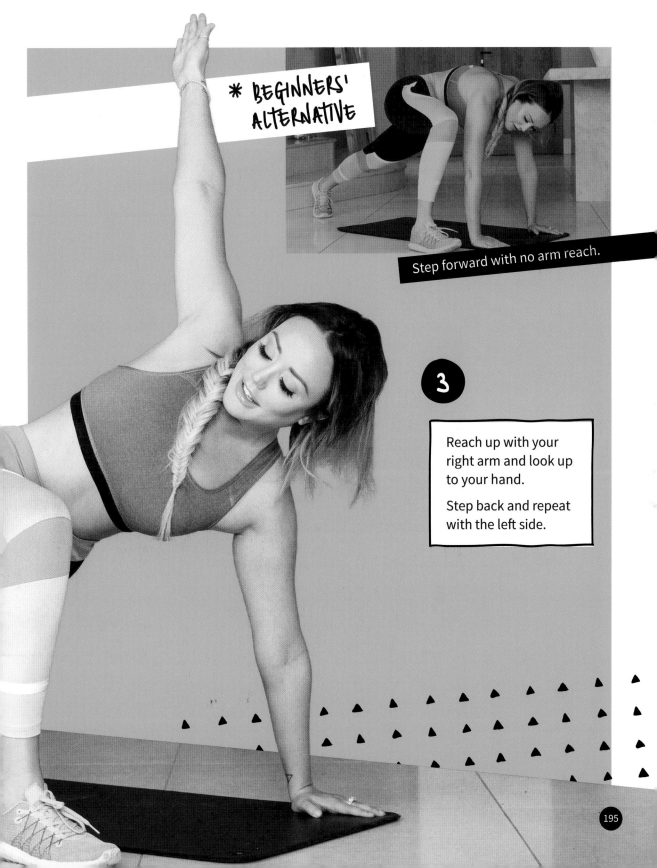

Step forward with no arm reach.

3

Reach up with your right arm and look up to your hand.

Step back and repeat with the left side.

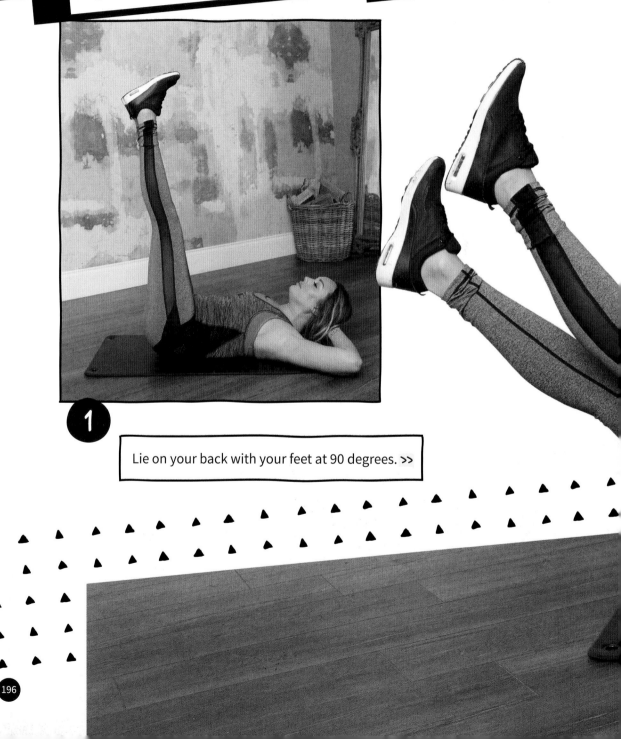

* SKYWALKERS

A killer ab exercise that looks super-cool.

1

Lie on your back with your feet at 90 degrees. >>

Plank. Hold in a press-up position.

2 Walk your feet down as far as you can maintaining straight legs, tight abs and keeping your back flat to the floor (imagine you are walking on an invisible path).

Then walk back up to the start position. **1**

197

* COWGIRL BURPEES

I love burpees – they're great... Love them or hate them, burpees are great for strength, fitness and fat-burning.

Start in a squat position and jump forward and back. **>>** **1**

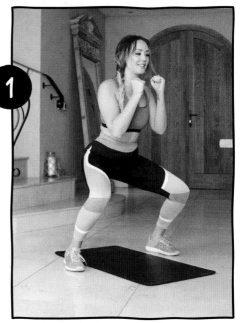

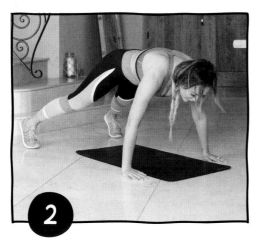

2

Keeping your feet wide, plant your hands flat to the floor and jump your feet back to a press-up position. Don't let your hips drop too low. **2** **>>**

Jump your feet forward. **>>** **3**

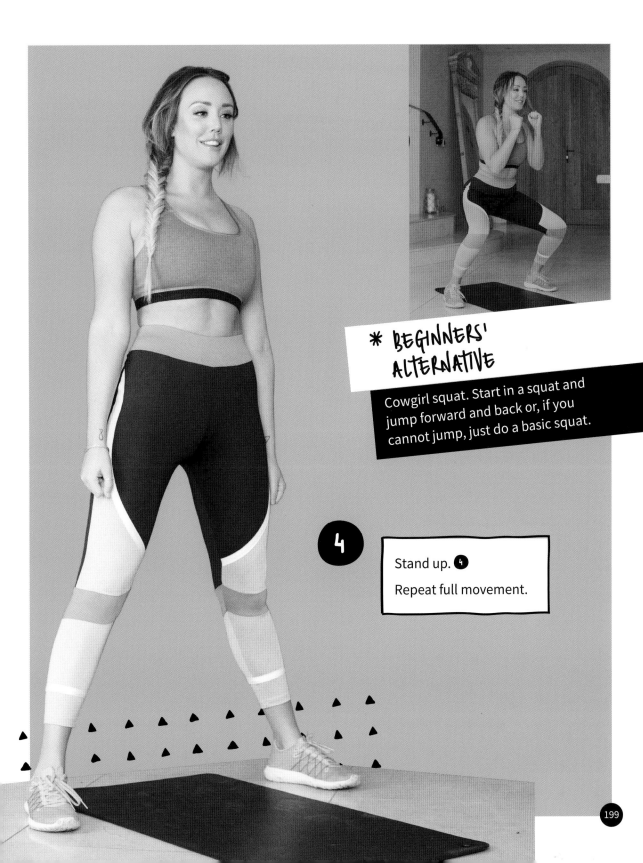

4

Stand up. **4**

Repeat full movement.

BOX KNEE & KICK OUT

You're really going to feel the burn with this bum-tightening and lifting exercise.

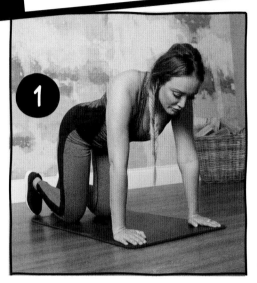

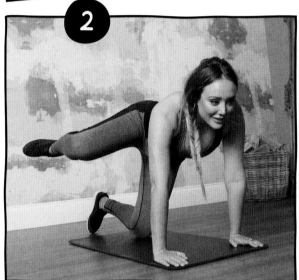

Begin in a box press-up position – hands under shoulders, knees under hips. >>

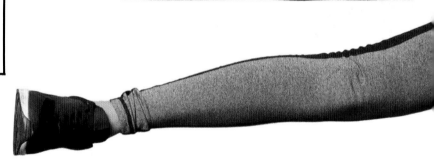

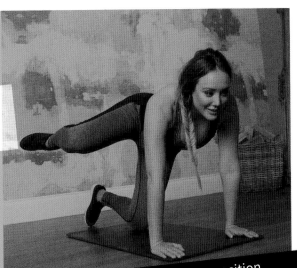

From box press-up position,
lift alternate knees up and down.

3

Maintain a 90-degree
angle at the knee joint
and lift your right knee
up and out to hip level
2 and then extend
your leg to the side. **3**

Reverse back to start
position. Repeat with
the left leg.

STAR JUMP & FRONT KICK

Have fun with this leg and ab fat burner.

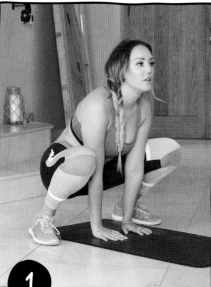

From a squat position ❶ jump in the air, reaching your arms as high and wide as possible and your legs as wide as possible. ❷

As you land, bend your knees to absorb the impact. »

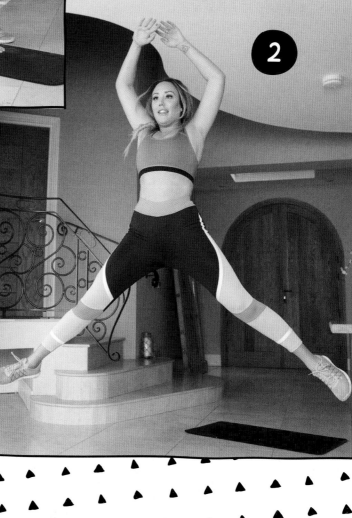

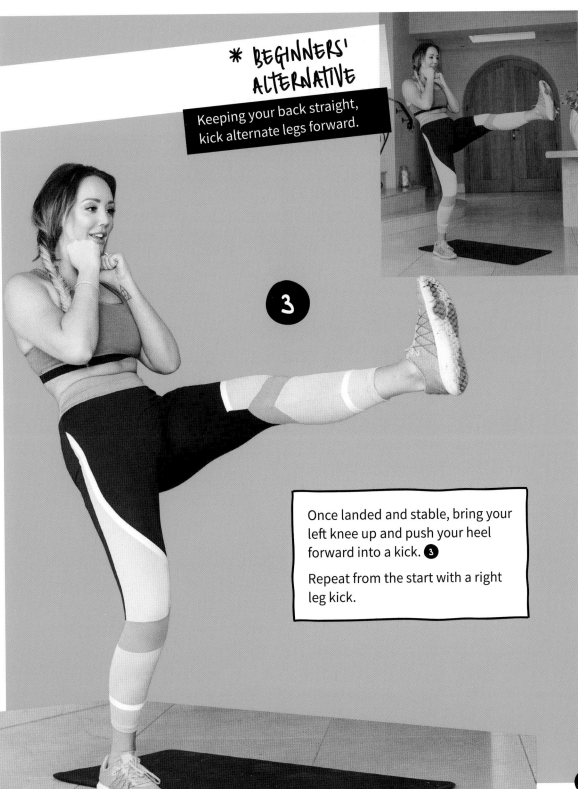

Keeping your back straight,
kick alternate legs forward.

3

Once landed and stable, bring your
left knee up and push your heel
forward into a kick. **3**

Repeat from the start with a right
leg kick.

CRUNCH & ALT KNEE

Another one for your abs – everyone loves a toned waist.

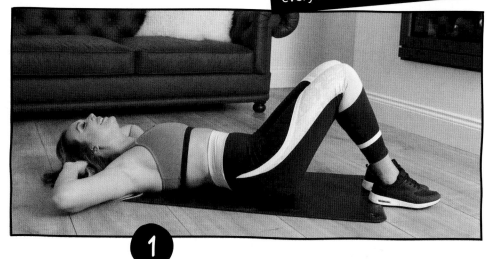

1

Lie on your back with your legs bent and feet flat. Put your fingertips to the back of the head to support the neck and look up rather than at your knees. ❶

Keeping your elbows wide and open, squeeze your abdominals – this is a crunch.

At the same time as you crunch, lift your left knee, ❷ lower and repeat with the right knee.

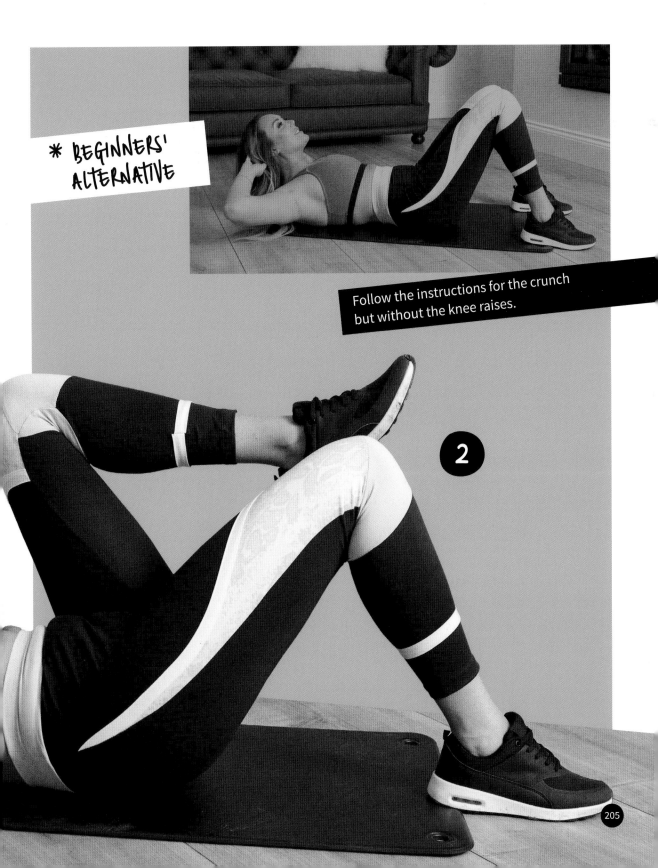

Follow the instructions for the crunch but without the knee raises.

2

✳ MOUNTAIN CLIMBERS

And *more* abs, with a bit of cardio thrown in.

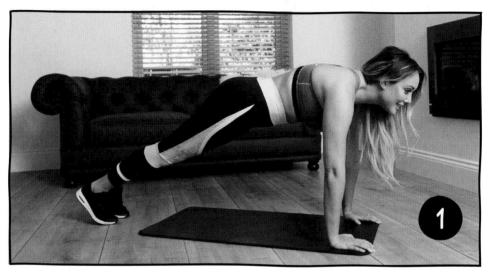

Start in a press-up position. ❶

With your shoulders staying over your hands, bring alternate knees as far forward as possible. ❷ Think about squeezing your abdominals on each climber.

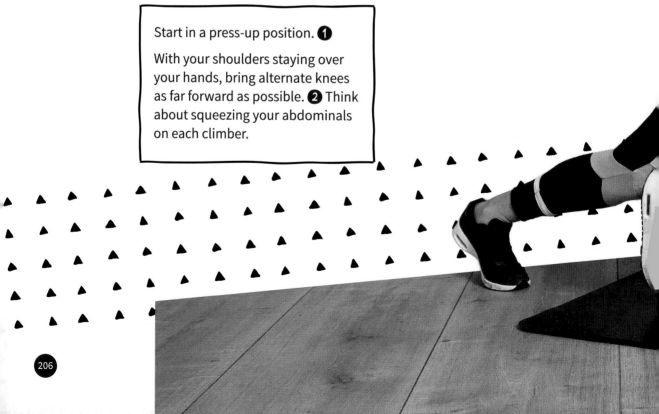

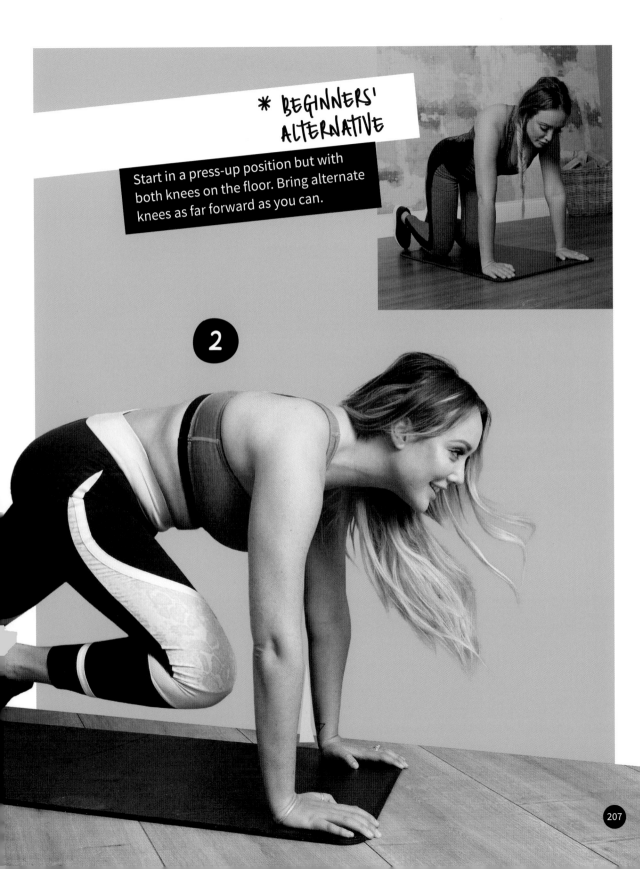

✱ BEGINNERS' ALTERNATIVE

Start in a press-up position but with both knees on the floor. Bring alternate knees as far forward as you can.

2

LATERAL JABS & JACKS

This combat sequence is a great stress-buster. Take that, stress!

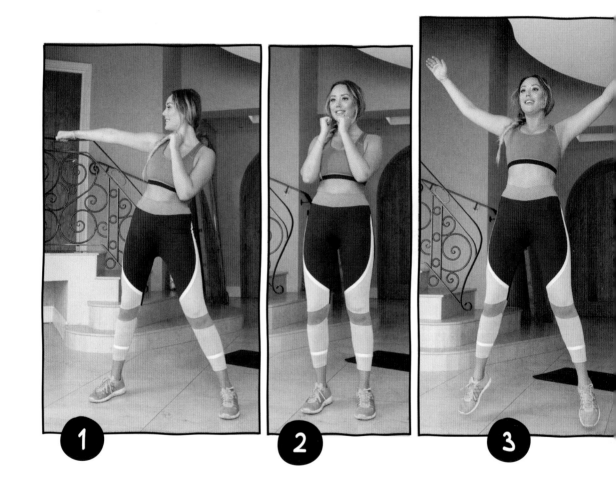

1

2

3

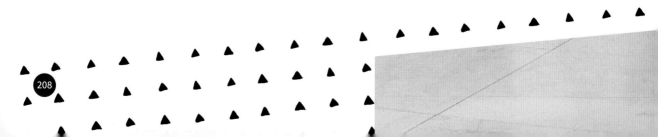

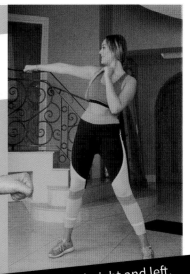

Side step out and side punch right and left.

4

Step or jump to the right side and extend your right arm into a side punch. **1**

Bring your feet back together **2** and then jump both feet wide and arms out, round and over your head into a jumping jack. **3**

Bring your feet together and arms down and repeat with the left side. **4**

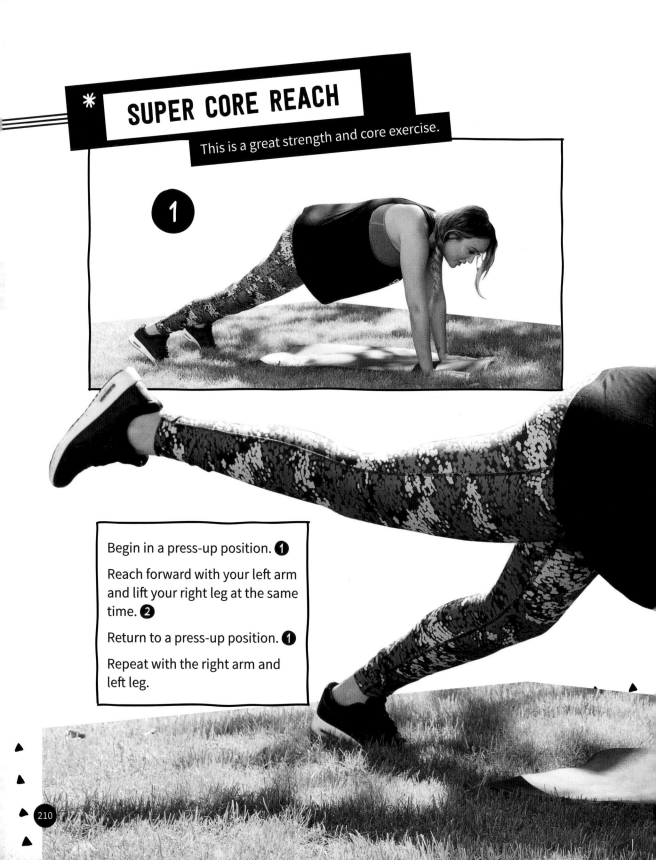

✳ SUPER CORE REACH

This is a great strength and core exercise.

1

Begin in a press-up position. **1**

Reach forward with your left arm and lift your right leg at the same time. **2**

Return to a press-up position. **1**

Repeat with the right arm and left leg.

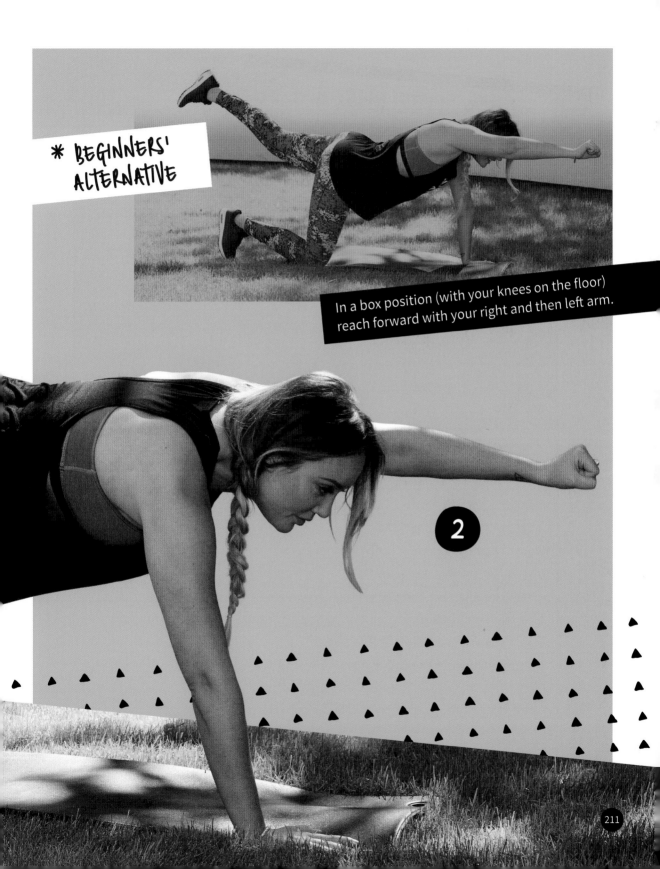

* BEGINNERS' ALTERNATIVE

In a box position (with your knees on the floor) reach forward with your right and then left arm.

2

ALTERNATE LUNGES & WOOD CHOPS

A thigh burner with a twist.

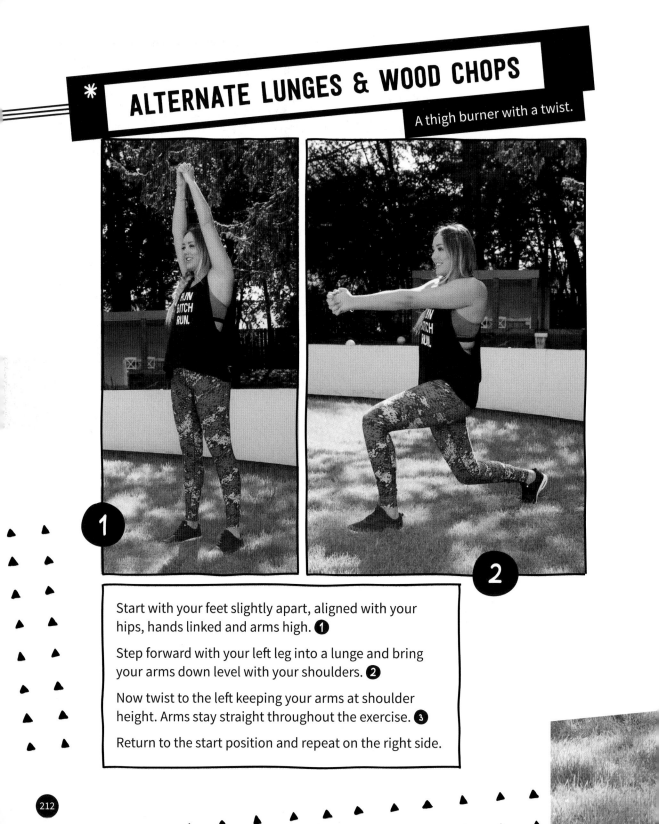

Start with your feet slightly apart, aligned with your hips, hands linked and arms high. **1**

Step forward with your left leg into a lunge and bring your arms down level with your shoulders. **2**

Now twist to the left keeping your arms at shoulder height. Arms stay straight throughout the exercise. **3**

Return to the start position and repeat on the right side.

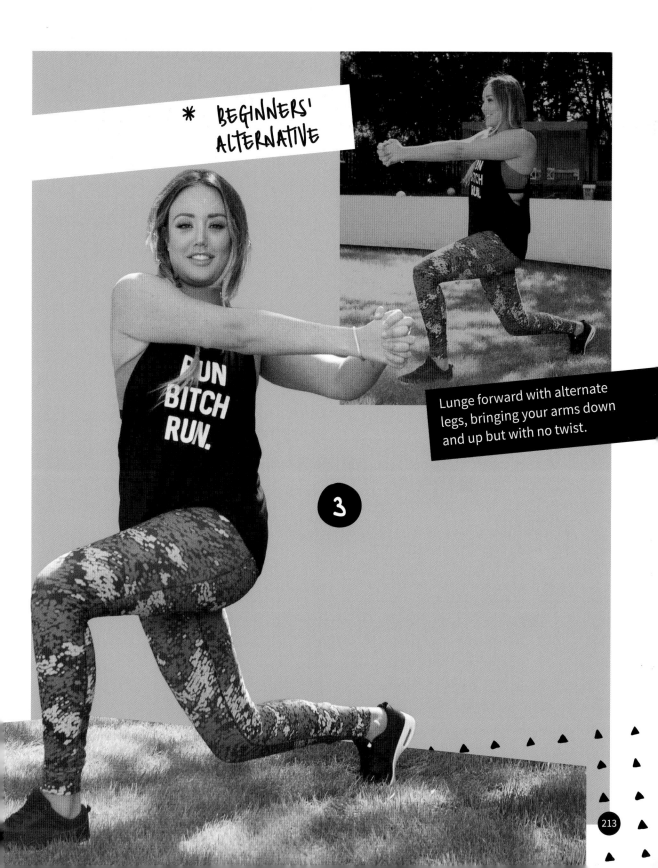

3

Lunge forward with alternate legs, bringing your arms down and up but with no twist.

STRETCHES &
COOL-DOWN

The hard work is done and now we want to slow things down and lower your heart rate. Your muscles will all be full and tight so you need to stretch them back to where they were before your workout. Hold each stretch for 10 to 15 seconds.

* STANDING BACK STRETCH

Link your hands together and push forward, stretching your shoulder blades apart.

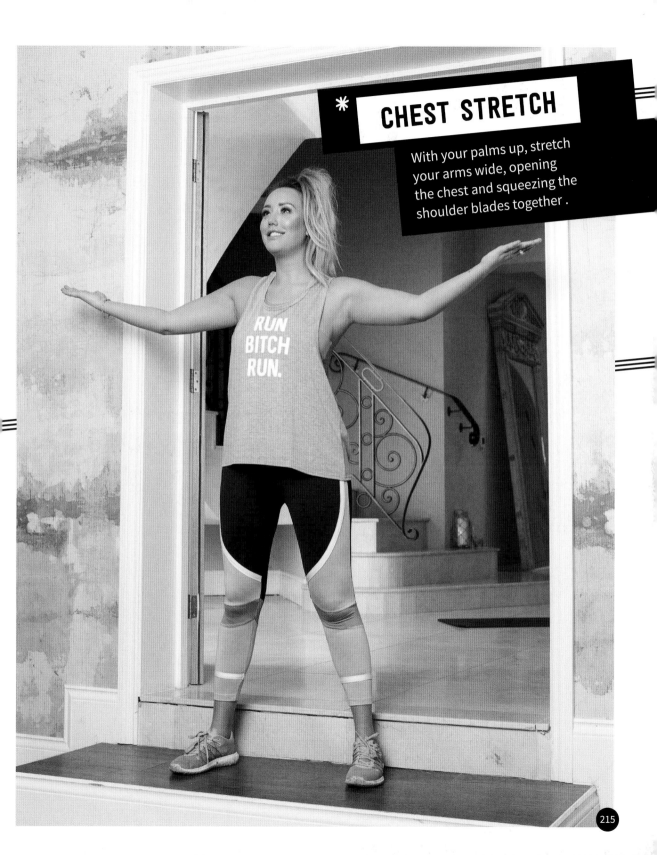

CHEST STRETCH

With your palms up, stretch your arms wide, opening the chest and squeezing the shoulder blades together .

CONT...

* OTT TRICEP STRETCH

Keeping your palms together, bend your arms behind the head and push your head back into your wrists/arms.

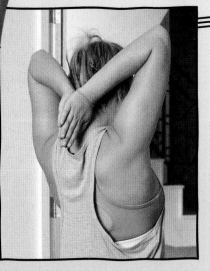

STANDING HAMSTRING STRETCH

Place your hands on the top of your thighs, step one foot forward and lean forward from the hips – maintain a straight back by opening the chest, squeezing the shoulder blades together and looking up. Repeat with the other leg.

QUAD STRETCH

Hold a chair or wall and grab your ankle and pull towards the butt. Try and keep the knees together. For an added stretch tilt the hip forwards. Repeat with the other leg.

NO SUCH THING AS CAN'T

So we've reached the end of the plan. How do you feel!!?? You should be SO IMPRESSED with yourself that you can't even look at your reflection in the mirror in case it STUNS you with its glory and beauty! I would like you to give yourself a great big fat (with a 'ph') pat on the back (the back that will now be feeling much more toned and muscular and won't ache so much because you haven't been slouching on it on the sofa like usual over the last month).

It's a massive achievement to get this far and even if you had a minor slip up you can forgive yourself because you committed to 30 days of challenges, new eating habits and moving your body about. I hope you feel as great inside as you look on the outside.

And I hope you now feel motivated and spurred on to keep it up and maintain some of the eating habits and exercises you've picked up along the way. You don't need to carry on doing it religiously every day but it should hopefully make you feel like you're in a zone and want to carry it on. Remember my other book – *Live Fast Lose Weight* – has loads of other recipes you can also follow if you want some variety. But keep this book and keep our Personal Trainer David too: in your pocket, on your bedside table and in your life because everyone needs a David in their lives forever!

In honour of you completing my 30-Day Blitz with me, I would like to finish by giving a shout-out to the 30 things I always put off and never do. I promise I will make it my resolution to do all of them now I've finished this book!

1. Make my bed every day.

2. Spend more time with the people I love.
I'm so lucky to be busy with so many brilliant work opportunities but it does mean I don't see my family or friends as much as I'd like.

3. Learn to spell.
The word 'exercise' is the hardest for me to get my head around – I always end up writing 'exsercise' (so it's a good job there is someone else checking the spellings in this book).

4. Finally watch *Game of Thrones*.
My mates ALL talk about it and I am left out. I tried to watch an episode once and wasn't concentrating enough so I didn't understand it and it washed right over me. I don't know any of the characters apart from the fact that Ed Sheeran was in it once.

5. Learn to play the piano.
I have always wanted to get one but I am convinced I wouldn't touch it and it would sit there and collect dust.

6. Have a meeting about my finances with my dad.

7. Tidy my bedroom.

8. Learn to sing and dance at the same time.
I have always wanted to be able to sing every Rhianna song in the world and gyrate like she does without falling off the bar.

9. Dog walking.

Take my dogs Rhubarb and Baby for their second walk of the day. WHY do they need two walks? I'll never understand. There is a garden for that.

10. Stop mixing my drinks.

And know when one more Jägerbomb is one too many Jägerbombs. Or Jägervoms.

11. Stop leaving my Tupperware everywhere.

It makes taking lunches with me a right ball-ache when I'm on my travels and have to buy a load more!

12. Unload the dishwasher instead of just getting things out of it when I need them.

13. Sign my name on all of my calendars.

I have to sign loads of them and by the end my name just looks like an alien squiggle. And my hand hurts. I need a magic arm to do the work for me!

14. Stop moaning so much about photo shoots (I hate them).

15. Never wear high heels again. ERGHHHHH!

16. Learn a language.

I'd quite like to learn Chinese because it's my favourite takeaway and then I could order it in the original language.

17. Learn to drive a bus.

Maybe I can have a super fancy tour bus one day and then I can drive it on my own!

18. Make me mam a cup of tea.

19. Actually do the things my agent asks me to do.

20. Watch the football so I can have a conversation about it with the men in my life.

21. Learn ballroom dancing so I can pretend I'm on *Strictly*.

22. Leave me mam nice notes around the house to tell her I love her.

23. See me brother Nathaniel more. I miss him when I'm away from him.

24. Run a marathon.

25. Wash my own hair.

How many other 27-year-olds still get their mam to do it for them?

26. Pay my phone bill.

27. Do the gardening.

I do not have green fingers. Nor do I want them. I like the colour of my fingers as they are (a sort of peachy tan). But I would like to know how to keep some of my plants and flowers alive, just in case they need me one day (and for when me mam or the gardener are on holiday).

28. Control my temper – especially with me mam.

29. Mop the floor.

30. Buy me mam flowers.

INDEX